THERAPEUTIC TAPING

FOR MUSCULOSKELETAL CONDITIONS

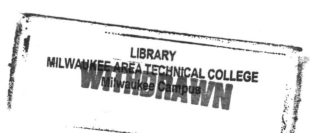

THERAPEUTIC TAPING

FOR MUSCULOSKELETAL CONDITIONS

Maria Constantinou

Mark Brown

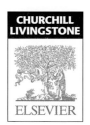

CHURCHILL
LIVINGSTONE

ELSEVIER

Sydney   Edinburgh   London   New York   Philadelphia   St Louis   Toronto

Churchill Livingstone
is an imprint of Elsevier

Elsevier Australia. ACN 001 002 357
(a division of Reed International Books Australia Pty Ltd)
Tower 1, 475 Victoria Avenue, Chatswood, NSW 2067

National Library of Australia Cataloguing-in-Publication Data

Author: Constantinou, Maria.
Title: Therapeutic taping for musculoskeletal conditions /
    Maria Constantinou & Mark Brown.
ISBN: 9780729539173 (pbk.)
Subjects: Musculoskeletal system--Diseases--Treatment.
    Musculoskeletal system--Wounds and injuries--Treatment.
Other Authors/Contributors: Brown, Mark.
Dewey Number: 612.7

Publisher: Melinda McEvoy
Developmental Editor: Sam McCulloch
Publishing Services Manager: Helena Klijn
Project Coordinator: Geraldine Minto
Edited by Forsyth Publishing Services
Proofread by Tim Learner
Cover, internal design and typesetting by Avril Makula
Illustrations by Lorenzo Lucia
Index by Forsyth Publishing Services
Printed by 1010 Printing International Ltd.

Contents

Foreword

In *Therapeutic Taping for Musculoskeletal Conditions*, Maria Constantinou and Mark Brown have produced a very comprehensive, practical and user-friendly text for clinicians and students from a range of disciplines. Physical therapists, athletic trainers, doctors, podiatrists, chiropractors, osteopaths and other musculoskeletal clinicians will find this book invaluable and one that will be used frequently in their practice — to gain new taping ideas, to refresh one's memory of particular techniques and to understand the current evidence.

This is a very practical book with an easy-to-use format. The book is organised in a clear and logical manner. The first three chapters provide an overview of therapeutic taping, its principles and effects as well as precautions and preparation procedures. The remaining chapters are arranged according to the anatomical region, covering the upper body, lower body and spine. At each region, a range of techniques have been compiled including those aimed at restricting range, deloading soft tissues, facilitating or inhibiting muscle activity, providing stability and support, and relieving pain. Soft casting is also covered as an alternative to taping for patients who may require ongoing taping or who are sensitive to adhesive tape.

For each taping technique the authors present a short background and rationale for its use, research evidence if available, material required, patient and therapist position, a detailed step-by-step application procedure with photographs and the use of relevant outcome measures for evaluation of the technique. The accompanying DVD is a valuable asset, particularly for those more complex techniques, reinforcing the taping application descriptions in the text. A sample standardised patient information sheet specifically designed for musculoskeletal taping is included in Appendix 2, and is a clinical tool that can be utilised by therapists.

A strength of the book is its inclusion and discussion of the research evidence (or lack thereof) for each taping technique. This is done in a thorough yet concise and useful manner to facilitate its relevance for clinicians. Appendix 1 provides a detailed table of the methodology and results of individual studies for those who wish to have a greater understanding of the research evidence for musculoskeletal taping.

In all, this is a user-friendly text which will find an important place in the clinic or office of the musculoskeletal practitioner, to be consulted on a regular basis.

Kim Bennell, PhD
Professor of Physiotherapy and Director
of the Centre for Health, Exercise
and Sports Medicine,
School of Health Sciences
University of Melbourne,
Melbourne, Australia

Authors

Maria Constantinou
MPhtySt(Sports) BPhty GradCerEd
FASMF
APA Sports Physiotherapist
Lecturer, School of Physiotherapy and
Exercise Science, Griffith Health Institute,
Griffith University, Australia

Mark Brown
MHSc(Sports Physio) BAppSc(Phty) MBA
FASMF
APA Sports Physiotherapist
Executive Officer Sports Medicine
Australia Queensland Branch, Australia
Assistant Professor of Physiotherapy,
School of Health Sciences and Medicine,
Bond University, Australia

Maria Constantinou and **Mark Brown**
are both Australian Physiotherapy
Association Sport Physiotherapists and
Fellows of the Australian Sports Medicine
Federation. Both have extensive clinical
experience in sports and musculoskeletal
physiotherapy, including major event
experience such as the Sydney 2000
Olympic Games, the Athens 2004
Olympic Games, the Melbourne 2006
Commonwealth Games and the
Vancouver 2010 Olympic Winter Games.

Reviewers

Michael Storr
B Physio
Lecturer, (Musculoskeletal) and Year
Level/Unit Coordinator — Physiotherapy
Department, Faculty of Medicine,
Nursing and Health Sciences, Monash
University, Victoria

Di Hopper
PhD(UWA); MEd(UWA);
BAppSc(Physio);
GradDipSportsPhysio(WAIT); FAMF;
APA Sports Physiotherapist titled member
Associate Professor, Curtin University of
Technology, School of Physiotherapy;
Postgraduate Coordinator, Western
Australia

Susan Gordon
PhD, BaAppSc(Physio)
Associate Professor, Discipline of
Physiotherapy, James Cook University,
Queensland

Acknowledgments

The techniques described in this book
have been selected by us from a range of
sources including discussions with
colleagues, courses attended, textbooks,
published literature and personal
innovation during our many years of
collective clinical and teaching experience
in a variety of settings. We wish to thank
all of our colleagues who were involved in
discussions on taping and who
contributed to our knowledge and
experience in these therapeutic taping
techniques and provided informal advice,
suggestions and support for this project.

We also would like to thank the many
reviewers who were involved in the
production of this book, and our
photography models for their time and
patience during the photo and DVD
shoot.

THERAPEUTIC TAPING

FOR MUSCULOSKELETAL CONDITIONS

CHAPTER 1
Introduction to therapeutic taping

This book aims to provide a practical guide to taping techniques used in the management of musculoskeletal conditions within a scientific framework. It is targeted at qualified and student physiotherapists, physical therapists, athletic trainers, doctors, podiatrists, chiropractors, osteopaths and other musculoskeletal clinicians.

WHAT IS THERAPEUTIC TAPING?

The Compact Oxford Dictionary (2009) defines 'therapeutic' as relating to the healing of disease, or having a good effect on the body or mind. Following this definition therapeutic taping techniques are techniques that utilise adhesive strapping tape as a component of the management of patients with musculoskeletal conditions.

The purpose of this book is to guide therapists on how to select and incorporate therapeutic taping techniques into clinical practice. Therapists have many clinical tools at their disposal and it is certainly not our contention that taping techniques are a panacea. However, they can be a useful component of the treatment for some musculoskeletal conditions.

Amongst other things, tape can be used clinically to reduce strain on damaged tissues, provide mechanical support to facilitate correct movement patterns, and facilitate or inhibit muscle activity. Used for these purposes, taping techniques can assist the therapist to address the underlying cause of a patient's condition. Taping techniques are rarely used in isolation, rather they are usually utilised in conjunction with appropriate exercises or other manual therapy techniques. The actual effects of taping as a therapeutic tool will be further explored in Chapter 2. Suggestions as to how the techniques can be utilised into clinical practice will be expanded upon under the description of each technique in Chapters 4, 5 and 6.

It should also be noted that as the book's focus is on therapeutic taping techniques, taping techniques intended for the purpose of injury prevention are not specifically covered (there are many texts already on that subject), but they are included and discussed where the same techniques also have a therapeutic purpose. There is a also a section in the literature review text in Chapter 2 that briefly examines the evidence in relation to the effectiveness of taping in injury prevention.

THE EVIDENCE-BASED APPROACH

The concept of utilising an evidence-based approach to clinical practice is now well established across most health professions. An aim of this book is to incorporate available evidence wherever possible while discussing the use of taping techniques for musculoskeletal conditions.

As stated by Hoffman, Bennett and Del Mar (2010), the purpose of evidence-based practice is to assist in clinical decision making and that for clinicians to be able to make informed clinical decisions many pieces of information need to be integrated. Herbert et al (2005) point out that high quality clinical research is not the only source of information that clinicians must take into account; rather, practice should also be informed by the professional knowledge of the therapist and, in addition, patient preferences.

Chapter 2 provides a summary of some of the available published evidence relating to the use of taping for musculoskeletal conditions. The main purpose of Chapter 2 is to provide the reader with an overview of some of the directions researchers have taken while trying to establish the effects and effectiveness of taping techniques as a treatment modality for musculoskeletal conditions. In this edition, we have not sought to undertake a comprehensive systematic review of the literature relating to taping. Rather, the purpose of the literature review is to inform clinicians as to the available evidence about some of the possible mechanisms that cause tape to be a useful clinical tool. With this information clinicians may be better able to adapt and incorporate the techniques to the specific needs of the patient, rather than follow a recipe approach to treatment.

Where research evidence for a technique exists, this will be discussed in the background and rationale section of each technique in Chapters 4, 5, 6 and 7.

The quality of research relating to taping varies widely. There are various systems describing levels of scientific evidence. Where appropriate, reference to levels of evidence discussed in this book is based on an adaptation of the classification system from the Australian National Health and Medical Research Council (NHMRC) (http://www.nhmrc.gov.au/index.htm), which is described in Table 1.1.

TABLE 1.1 LEVELS OF EVIDENCE (NATIONAL HEALTH AND MEDICAL RESEARCH COUNCIL)

LEVEL OF EVIDENCE	STUDY DESIGN
I	Evidence obtained from a systematic review of all relevant randomised controlled trials.
II	Evidence obtained from at least one properly designed randomised controlled trial.
III-1	Evidence obtained from well-designed pseudo-randomised controlled trials (alternate allocation or some other method).
III-2	Evidence obtained from comparative studies (including systematic reviews of such studies) with concurrent controls and allocation not randomised, cohort studies, case-control studies, or interrupted time series with a control group.
III-3	Evidence obtained from comparative studies with historical control, two or more single-arm studies, or interrupted time series without a parallel control group.
IV	Evidence obtained from case series, either post test or pre-test/post test.

Clinical or case reports are not part of the NHMRC levels of evidence classification system. However, in the absence of higher levels of evidence, clinical decision making may be based on clinical or case reports. These are described in some classification systems such as the Oxford Centre for Evidence Based Medicine (CEBM) levels of evidence as Level V (http://www.cebm.net/index.aspx?o=1025, accessed 29 March 2010). When discussing clinical or case reports in context of the therapeutic taping techniques described in this book they will be referred to as either clinical or case reports.

Given the varying quality of, or in some cases the lack of, published scientific research for some of the taping techniques, the use of appropriate outcome measures which can provide the patient and therapist with a clear indication of the effectiveness of the technique are necessary. Outcome measures can also assist the therapist to make evidence-based informed decisions, including in determining the effectiveness of modified or innovative techniques that in their professional judgment may be more appropriate for a particular patient or types of patient.

OUTCOME MEASURES USED IN CLINICAL PRACTICE PERTAINING TO TAPING

Appropriate outcome measures, which are tests or scales used to measure function or performance of patients at a point in time, are a necessity in patient management in any health care setting. Measures of outcomes can also be used to evaluate change of the patient's condition or function over time, by looking at the difference from one point in time (before an intervention or at the initial assessment session) to another point in time (following an intervention or at a follow-up assessment session). Outcome measures utilised in a musculoskeletal clinical setting can be of subjective nature, they may include measures of objective or functional tests, or the use of validated questionnaires specific to the patient's condition, presentation or goals. Discussion and critical evaluation of different outcome measures used in a musculoskeletal clinical setting is a stand-alone topic and it is beyond the scope of this book. However, it is important throughout this book that the reader considers the use of outcome measures to evaluate the indication and efficacy of therapeutic taping techniques.

The subjective examination or history taking is an integral part of the patient consultation process and gives the therapist an insight into the description, behaviour and intensity of the patient's symptoms, functional limitations and goals of treatment. This information contributes to the clinical reasoning process and assists in developing an effective patient-centred management approach, which includes use of relevant and specific outcome measures. Identified relevant outcome measures may be used before and/or after the application of therapeutic techniques, including taping, to evaluate the indication and efficacy of each technique.

The most common clinical outcome measures referred to in this book in the evaluation of therapeutic taping techniques are:

1 Pain free active range of motion (ROM) is a commonly used outcome measure in musculoskeletal assessment and can be measured using various goniometric methods. Some commonly used goniometric tools are described below.

   a A standard goniometer can be used to measure ROM in most joints in the body. The goniometer has been shown to have a good intratester reliability within 2°–3° and fair to good intertester reliability within 5°–6° (Rothstein, Miller & Roettger 1983). Goniometric measurements of ROM have been studied in a variety of body regions and have been found to be reliable within a 2°–5° range (Edgar et al 2009).

   b A fluid filled plurimeter measures ROM in certain body regions. A plurimeter is an instrument with incremental markings on a dial that rotates to measure the angle ROM of one body area relative to another. A plurimeter can be used as an alternative to a goniometer, as for instance, in the measure of hip internal and external rotation (Croft et al 1996) or in cervical spine flexion and extension.

   c An inclinometer is a mechanical or electronic device which measures the relative inclination of a body area with respect to gravity. Generally two sensors are required to be used concurrently, one of which is stationary and the other is attached to the moving body part and records the reference of one point to the other. An example of the use of an inclinometer is in the measurement of cervical spine flexion ROM (Antonaci et al 2000) or lumbar spine ROM (Chen et al 1997).

  d A standard soft tape measure may be used when measuring ROM in certain body areas, such as the lumbar spine (Fitzgerald et al 1983).

2 There are three main pain rating scales commonly used to evaluate the perception of pain.

  a The visual analogue scale (VAS) which uses a 10 cm blank line (Fig 1.1). The patient is asked to record their pain level on the line where one end is indicative of 'no pain at all' and the other end is indicative of the 'worst imaginable pain'. This scale needs to be delivered in a written format and consistency in its delivery – to being in either a horizontal or a vertical line – is necessary (Williamson & Hoggart 2005), with the horizontal line being most commonly used. The clinically significant change is thought to be at 30–33% difference in the pain rate (Williamson & Hoggart 2005).

  b The numerical rating scale (Fig 1.2) requires the patient to record their pain level by circling a number from 0–10 on a 10 cm line with 1 cm increments from zero (0) 'no pain at all' to ten (10) 'worst imaginable pain'. This scale can be delivered verbally or in a written format (Williamson & Hoggart 2005). A reduction of two points or 30% change is considered a clinically meaningful change (Farrar et al 2001).

  c The verbal rating scale is a process whereby the patient is asked to describe their pain level on a list of incremental adjectives such as, for instance, 'no pain; mild pain; moderate pain; and severe or intense pain' which are assigned a numerical value from 0–3 (Williamson & Hoggart 2005).

All three pain rating scales have been found to be valid clinical measures, particularly when used within the same patient comparison (Maxwell 1978; Williamson & Hoggart 2005). It is important to note that the use of these scales can be applied by the patient when describing the intensity of their pain at rest, and/or during active ROM, or during a nominated functional task. For instance, the pain level on the lateral hip area may be rated by the patient during rest, during active hip

No pain at all —————————————————————————————— Worst pain imaginable

FIGURE 1.1 THE VISUAL ANALOGUE SCALE (VAS)

O_____1_____2_____3_____4_____5_____6_____7_____8_____9_____10

No pain   Worst imaginable pain

FIGURE 1.2 THE NUMERICAL RATING SCALE

flexion and then compared during walking and during stair climbing, before and after the use of a hip application taping technique.

3 The patient specific functional scale (PSFS) requires that the therapist asks the patient during the subjective or history taking session 'Today, are there any activities that you are unable to do or having difficulty with because of your [nominated] problem?' (Sterling & Brentnall 2007). The patient is asked to nominate three main activities they have difficulty performing and to rate each of these activities on an 11-point scale (0–10), where zero (0) is 'Unable to perform activity at all' and ten (10) is 'Able to perform activity at the pre-injury or problem level' (Westaway, Stratford & Binkley 1998). This scale has the capacity to measure change over time and has been shown to have a minimal detectable change value of two points when the average score of the three activities is used and three points for each single activity score. The validity and sensitivity of the PSFS change has been demonstrated in several musculoskeletal conditions such as cervical radiculopathy (Cleland et al 2006), neck (Westaway et al 1998) and low back pain (Pengel, Refshauge & Maher 2004), in patients with knee pain (Chatman et al 1997) and in functional limitation of patients with work-related injuries (Gross, Battie & Asante 2008). The PSFS is available in a simple form which is easy to apply and is available at the time of writing on the Transit Accident Commission of Victoria website, accessed through: http://www.workcover.vic.gov.au/wps/wcm/resources/file/eb5b3b42810d1fd/patient_specific.pdf

When making an informed decision regarding the therapeutic effect of a taping technique the therapist needs to be aware what change constitutes a minimum detectable difference. In the application of taping, a clinical change commonly employed by therapists is improvement of 50% or better in the symptoms being addressed with tape (McConnell 2002; Vicenzino et al 2008). This is supported by Farrar et al (2001) who found a change of 50% or more in the numerical scale could represent a 'very much improved' verbal rating. However, as suggested by Rowbotham (2001) in his editorial 'What is a "clinically meaningful" reduction in pain', a value of 30% reduction in numerical rating could represent a 'much improved' verbal rating and it could be regarded as a meaningful clinical improvement.

ANATOMY KNOWLEDGE

Excellent knowledge of anatomy of the area to be taped is imperative to the success of the technique and the safety of the patient. An assumed level of anatomy knowledge by the therapist is expected in the application of the techniques described in this book. If uncertain, the therapist needs to ensure they review the anatomical details of the area to be taped in preparation. It is beyond the scope of this book to provide a detailed anatomical description of each area to be taped, but it is hoped that a comprehensive musculoskeletal anatomy book may be utilised as a reference where necessary during the application of taping.

TERMS AND DEFINITIONS

This book aims to have a consistent language approach used throughout. It is important for the reader to be aware that, unless otherwise stated, throughout this book the following applies:

1 All references to athletes, patients and clients are confined to the use of the word 'patient'.

2 All references to the physical therapist, physiotherapist, athletic trainer and other clinicians are confined to the use of the word 'therapist'.

3 The word 'tape' or 'taping' will be used to refer to 38 mm width adhesive rigid tape, which is considered to be the most commonly used tape (Bragg et al 2002).

4 The word 'hypoallergenic underlay' will be used to refer to tape that is hypoallergenic, perforated, and elastic in its width but not length. In this book 5 cm width hypoallergenic underlay is used.

5 The use of the term 'range of motion' will be abbreviated as ROM.

6 The use of the word 'centimetre' will be confined to the common abbreviation 'cm'.

7 The use of the term 'lumbrical grip' will be used to refer to the therapist's position of metacarpophalangeal flexion of fingers 1 up to 4 (which use the lumbrical muscle action) and the thumb position of carpometacarpal adduction and metacarpophalangeal flexion, as the thumb and fingers come together to grip during the application of a manual therapy technique.

The reader should also consider the following important points during the application of the therapeutic taping techniques.

1 The use of hypoallergenic underlay will be described where it is an integral part of the technique. However, its use is not limited to those techniques alone and the therapist may opt to use it with other techniques.

2 The use of elasticised adhesive bandage may be used over taping techniques to reinforce the application of tape if desired, or if the patient plans to perform vigorous activities after the application of the taping technique.

3 An explanation should be given to the patient describing the purpose of each technique, and informed consent should be gained each time the technique is applied.

4 A standard warning regarding taping precautions is described in Chapter 3, and this should be given after each tape application. When a more specific warning is relevant to a particular technique, over and above the standard warning described in Chapter 3, it will be included at the end of each technique.

5 After the application of each taping technique an evaluation of the effectiveness of the technique needs to be performed using appropriate outcome measures. Some possible outcome measures are described at the completion of each taping technique. However, these are only a guide and the therapist may choose to use other specific outcomes relevant to the patient and/or condition being treated.

HOW THIS BOOK IS STRUCTURED

This book is structured so that the reader reviews Chapters 1–3 to gain the relevant background information that relates to the use of taping as a therapeutic tool prior to reading Chapters 4–6, which relate to the application of therapeutic taping techniques to specific body regions. Chapter 7 describes a sampler of soft casting techniques which can be used in place of taping for certain patients who require ongoing taping and/or are sensitive to the adhesive material used in the manufacture of taping. Each taping technique described in Chapters 4–7 is a stand-alone technique starting on a separate page and includes background and rationale for its use, material required, patient and therapist position, step-by-step application procedures with photographs and the use of relevant outcome measures for evaluation of the technique. The therapist, whether a student or an experienced clinician, is able to utilise as much or as little of the information provided for each taping technique to apply the technique effectively.

The structure of the book is as follows:

Chapter 1 • Introduction

This chapter introduces therapeutic taping and provides an overview of the approach the book will take, including how the evidence is discussed, the use of outcome measures in the application of taping and common terms and definitions employed throughout the book.

Chapter 2 • Review of the principles and effects

Chapter 2 reviews available evidence in the literature on the use of taping, and discusses the general effects of taping for musculoskeletal conditions.

Chapter 3 • Precautions and preparation procedures

The general and specific precautions and contraindications to taping are discussed in this chapter. Furthermore, this chapter outlines the general procedures for preparation of taping and the necessity of gaining informed consent prior to, and providing a precautionary warning after, the application of the taping technique.

Chapter 4 • Taping for musculoskeletal conditions of the upper body

Chapter 4 describes the application of taping techniques to the upper quadrant, which include scapula and postural taping, taping to the glenohumeral, acromioclavicular, elbow and wrist joints, and taping to the hand and fingers.

Chapter 5 • Taping for musculoskeletal conditions of the lower body

Chapter 5 describes the application of taping techniques to the lower quadrant, which include the hip, knee, tibiofibular and ankle joints and taping to the foot and toes.

Chapter 6 • Spinal conditions of cervical, thoracic and lumbar spine, pelvis and sacroiliac joint (SIJ)

Chapter 6 describes the application of taping techniques to the cervical, thoracic and lumbar spine, and to the pelvis and sacroiliac joints.

Chapter 7 • Soft casting techniques

Chapter 7 provides a sample of three soft casting techniques which can be used as an alternative to taping for patients who may require ongoing taping or who may develop, or are sensitive to, the adhesive material on tape. The techniques described in Chapter 7 are for soft casting to the thumb, ankle and foot.

Appendices

Appendix I contains a summary table of the most relevant research evidence relating to techniques described in this book. Appendix II contains a sample standardised patient information sheet, with warning and consent forms that may be utilised by therapists when using the therapeutic taping techniques described in this book.

REFERENCES

Antonaci, F, Ghirmai, S, Bono, G, Nappi, G (2000) Current methods for cervical spine movement evaluation: a review. Clinical and Experimental Rheumatology, 18(2): S45–S52.

Bragg, R W, MacMahon, J M, Overom, E K, Yerby, S A, Matheson, G O, Carter, D R, Andriacchi, T P (2002) Failure and fatigue characteristics of adhesive athletic tape. Medicine and Science in Sports and Exercise, 34(3): 403–10.

Chatman, A B, Hyams, S P, Neel, J M, Binkley, J M, Stratford, P W, Schomberg, A, Stabler, M (1997) The patient-specific functional scale: measurement properties in patients with knee dysfunction. Physical Therapy, 77(8): 820–9.

Chen, S C, Samo, D G, Chen, E H, Crampton, A R, Conrad, K M, Egan, L, Mitton, J (1997) Reliability of three lumbar sagittal motion measurement methods: surface inclinometers. Journal of Occupational and Environmental Medicine, 39(3): 217–23.

Cleland, J, Fritz, J, Whitman, J, Palmer, J (2006) The reliability and construct validity of the Neck Disability Index and patient specific functional scale in patients with cervical radiculopathy. Spine, 31(5): 598–602.

Compact Oxford English Dictionary. Online. Available: www.askoxford.com (accessed 2 Oct 2009).

Croft, P R, Nahit, E S, Macfarlane, G J, Silman, A J (1996) Interobserver reliability in measuring flexion, internal rotation, and external rotation of the hip using a plurimeter. Ann Rheum Dis, 55(5): 320–3.

Edgar, D, Finlay, V, Wu, A, Wood, F (2009) Goniometry and linear assessments to monitor movement outcomes: are they reliable tools in burn survivors? Burns, 35(1): 58–62.

Farrar, J T, Young, J P, LaMoreaux, L, Werth, J L, Poole, R M (2001) Clinical importance of changes in chronic pain intensity measured on an 11-point numerical pain rating scale. Pain, 94(2): 149–58.

Fitzgerald, G K, Wynveen, K J, Rheault, W, Rothschild, B (1983) Objective assessment with establishment of normal values for lumbar spinal range of motion. Physical Therapy, 63(11): 1776–81.

Gross, D P, Battie, M C, Asante, A K (2008) The Patient-Specific Functional Scale: validity in workers' compensation claimants. Archives of Physical Medicine and Rehabilitation, 89(7): 1294–9.

Herbert, R D, Jamtvedt, G, Mead, J, Birger Hagen, K (2005) Practical Evidence-Based Physiotherapy. Elsevier Australia, Sydney.

Hoffmann, T, Bennett, S, Del Mar, C (2010) Evidence-Based Practice Across the Health Professions. Elsevier Australia, Sydney.

Maxwell, C (1978) Sensitivity and accuracy of the Visual Analogue Scale: a psycho-physical classroom experiment. The British Journal of Clinical Pharmacology, 6(1): 15–24.

McConnell, J (2002) Recalcitrant chronic low back and leg pain — a new theory and different approach to management. Manual Therapy, 7(4): 183–92.

Pengel, L H M, Refshauge, K M, Maher, C G (2004) Responsiveness of pain, disability, and physical impairment outcomes in patients with low back pain. Spine, 29(8): 879–83.

Rothstein, J M, Miller, P J, Roettger, R F (1983) Goniometric reliability in a clinical setting: elbow and knee measurements. Physical Therapy 63(10): 1611–15.

Rowbotham, M C (2001) What is a 'clinically meaningful' reduction in pain? Pain 94(2): 131–2.

Sterling, M, Brentnall, D (2007) Patient Specific Functional Scale. Australian Journal of Physiotherapy, 53(1): 65.

Vicenzino, B, Collins, N, Crossley, K, Beller, E, Darnell, R, McPoil, T (2008) Foot orthoses and physiotherapy in the treatment of patellofemoral pain syndrome: a randomised clinical trial. BMC Musculoskeletal Disorders, 9, article 27.

Westaway, M D, Stratford, P W, Binkley, J M (1998) The patient-specific functional scale: validation of its use in persons with neck dysfunction. Journal of Orthopaedic and Sports Physical Therapy, 27(5): 331–8.

Williamson, A, Hoggart, B (2005) Pain: a review of three commonly used pain rating scales. Journal of Clinical Nursing, 14(7): 798–804.

CHAPTER 2

Review of the principles and effects

INTRODUCTION

In this book we have set out to provide a set of techniques that utilise therapeutic taping as an adjunct to treatment for various musculoskeletal conditions. This chapter summarises some of the significant published research related to the use of taping techniques. While all of the techniques in this book have been used clinically and with anecdotal or clinically observed positive outcomes associated with their use, only a comparatively small number have been explicitly examined in well-conducted published research studies. However, as much as has been possible with the current evidence, we have attempted to produce this book with an evidence-informed approach, utilising the highest levels of evidence where possible, and sound clinical rationale and reasoning for techniques without published evidence. It is our hope that the gaps in the evidence serve as a stimulus for further research and refinement of knowledge which will in turn result in a stronger evidence-based approach.

HISTORY OF THERAPEUTIC TAPING FOR MUSCULOSKELETAL CONDITIONS IN THE LITERATURE

Documented use of adhesive strapping tape as an adjunct to medical treatment goes back to at least as early as 1895 when Dr Virgil Gibney published an article in the *New York Medical Journal* titled 'Sprained ankle: a treatment that involves no loss of time, requires no crutches, and is not attended with an ultimate impairment of function' (Gibney 1895). In this article the author described a basket weave technique using strips of adhesive plaster as a treatment for ankle sprains.

In 1940 Walter Galland published an article in the *Journal of Bone and Joint Surgery* in which he carefully described a technique that was based on the 'Gibney boot', as he called the technique described by Gibney, but augmented by additional oblique strips of tape with the aim of limiting lateral movements of the calcaneum into either supination or pronation (Fig 2.1). His evidence for the described technique's superiority to the original Gibney basket weave taping was limited to a well-reasoned argument that limiting lateral calcaneal motion would reduce the strain on the injured calcaneofibular or calcaneotibial ligaments, and further supported 'on the basis of long experience with this dressing' (Galland 1940).

According to Berkowitz and Bottoni (2006) Gibney's basket weave technique described in 1895 subsequently found more

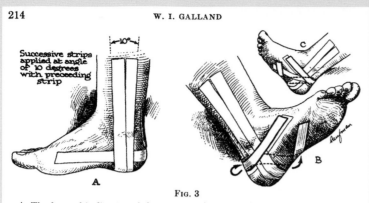

FIG. 3

A: The forward inclination of the successive longitudinal straps is illustrated. This inclination is necessary in order to have the straps conform naturally to the contour of the foot without wrinkling.

B and *C:* The interlocking of the first pair of horizontal straps is illustrated. The dotted lines indicate the location of the strap as it rounds the opposite side of the foot. It is the interlocking of these straps which produces the immobilization of the sub-astragalar articulations.

FIGURE 2.1 A DIAGRAM AND EXPLANATORY TEXT FROM THE ARTICLE BY GALLAND (1940)

widespread use as a method of injury prevention, though when this practice started is not clear from the available literature. However, the use of taping and bandages to protect the wrist and fingers of boxers was definitely well established by the early 1900s as evidenced by several contemporary photographs. Advertisements for strapping tape directed to American footballers appeared in the 1930s so the use of taping and strapping as an injury prevention technique in sports does appear to have gained rapid acceptance, which has continued until the present day.

However, while taping for acute injury management and injury prevention has been used by physical therapists/physiotherapists,

athletic trainers and sports trainers for many years, published research for its effectiveness as an adjunct to treatment is limited up until 1986.

In 1986 Jenny McConnell published an article titled 'The management of chondromalacia patellae: a long term solution' (McConnell 1986) in which the author described the use of a taping technique to correct the alignment of the patella, for the twofold purpose of reducing patellofemoral pain, and also for facilitating the action of the vastus medialis as a long-term solution for correction of one of the underlying causes of patellofemoral pain.

This novel approach to treatment precipitated the publication of several articles that sought to investigate the effectiveness of adhesive tape as an adjunct therapeutic tool in the management of a range of musculoskeletal conditions. As a result, an increasingly large catalogue of taping techniques for musculoskeletal conditions is now available to the therapist, some of which are well supported by a sound evidence base. As mentioned above, while the scientific evidence supporting the techniques in this book varies, it is our hope that the gaps in the evidence serve as a stimulus for further research and refinement of an even stronger evidence-based approach.

LITERATURE REVIEW OF THE EFFECTS OF TAPING AND THE CURRENT EVIDENCE

As mentioned in the introduction, the primary aim of this chapter is to summarise the evidence relating to the known and proposed effects of adhesive tape as a therapeutic tool. For this purpose an extensive literature review was conducted with the goal of identifying studies that have utilised taping or strapping in the management of musculoskeletal conditions. Databases searched included the Cochrane Library, the Physiotherapy Evidence Database (PEDro), Medline, Ovid, Pubmed, Scopus and SportDiscus. The main keywords searched were 'tape, taped, taping, strap, strapped, strapping, brace, braced, bracing' as well as various other search terms specific to the treatment of injuries and conditions that commonly involve taping as a component of treatment. In addition, a manual search of articles referenced by other authors was also undertaken.

The abstracts of the articles identified in the search were reviewed and articles relevant to therapeutic taping for musculoskeletal conditions were obtained in full. All papers of relevance were further reviewed and a summary of the main applicable findings of the key studies are included in this literature review. In addition, the relevant papers pertaining to region-specific techniques are included in the 'Evidence' section of each technique in Chapters 4–6.

While reading the review of the evidence on taping discussed in this and subsequent chapters the reader should bear in mind that although a multitude of studies were identified, there is still a need for more high quality research related to the use of tape as a therapeutic tool. While we identified several hundred relevant studies it is apparent that:

○ the quality of the published research varies widely
○ many of the conclusions were compromised by factors such as poor research design, inadequate description or standardisation of the techniques examined, or small sample numbers
○ even in the case of well-designed studies it is difficult to compare many of the outcomes because of a lack of uniformity of the techniques used between different research studies.

In addition, more research is required into the reproducibility and accuracy of the application of taping techniques, as well as any effects associated with the skill level and experience of the therapist applying the techniques.

In the pages that follow we will discuss some of the studies identified in the literature review. Also, at the end of the book we have included Appendix 1, a summary of the literature that directly relates to taping techniques described in Chapters 4–6. The purpose of this table is to give the reader the opportunity to identify the extent and quality of the available research that relates to each of the techniques described in this book.

THE INTENDED PURPOSES AND POSSIBLE EFFECTS OF TAPING TECHNIQUES

The studies identified in the literature review that describe the intended purposes and effects of tape can be broadly grouped into the following main categories:

1 pain reduction
2 injury or re-injury prevention
3 reduction of strain on injured or vulnerable tissues
4 provision of increased passive stability of anatomical structures
5 biomechanical correction
6 muscle inhibition
7 muscle facilitation

8 enhancement of proprioception

9 compression for oedema, or lymphatic drainage.

Some of these intended purposes could be achieved as a result of a combination of the following broadly described possible effects of tape:

1 mechanical effects

2 neuromuscular effects

3 psychological effects.

The following sections in this chapter discuss some of the findings identified in the literature review that relate to some of these categories and effects.

PAIN REDUCTION

Pain is one of the most frequent reasons patients present to therapists for treatment. Several studies have concluded that tape as an adjunct to treatment of musculoskeletal conditions does effectively decrease pain. If a therapist can reduce pain with tape it provides an opportunity to more adequately direct treatment to removal of the underlying causes of the condition.

However, the mechanism, or mechanisms, as to how tape assists in pain reduction is not fully established, but is likely related to a reduction of the stress on injured or pain-provoking tissues by the mechanical or neuromuscular effects of tape, which are described in more detail in the sections below.

Mechanical effects

Many of the proposed benefits or effects of taping for musculoskeletal conditions are based on mechanical principles. In this category joint support, joint re-alignment and biomechanical correction are all proposed benefits of taping.

Reduction of the strain on injured structures is one of the most basic propositions of the usefulness of taping in both the acute phase and also during ongoing repair and rehabilitation. Supporting an injured joint with tape is widely believed to be helpful in reducing pain, preventing exacerbation of the injury and promoting tissue healing (Shapiro et al 1994).

Many of the studies that examine the mechanical advantages that tape bestows advocate the use of tape for the purpose of injury or re-injury prevention, especially in sport. Tape is proposed to provide an external support to joints under load, and on this basis it is often applied to provide limitation to the movements or positions where the structures it is designed to protect are vulnerable. If the tape is applied with consideration to preventing extremes of normal joint movement its action can be compared to that of an external ligament (McLean 1989).

A number of researchers have sought to establish the degree to which strapping tape can actually cause definite effects on the biomechanics of the area taped. For example, Crossley et al (2009) conducted a study using magnetic resonance imaging (MRI) with patients with patella femoral joint osteoarthritis and found that tape produced a significant reduction in both lateral patella position and lateral patella tilt. These authors also found that the tape also reduced pain during squatting. Similarly, Larsen et al (1995) conducted a radiological study on the McConnell medial patella glide technique and found that glide and tape technique was effective in producing medial translation of the patella in most subjects; however, they also reported that tape was not able to maintain this position effectively after exercise. This was a very similar result to the findings of Pfeiffer et al (2004) who found that medial patella glide taping resulted in significant medial displacement at four knee angles before, but not after, exercise.

By contrast, Bockrath et al (1993) concluded from their X-ray study that while medial patella taping does decrease symptoms of patellofemoral pain syndrome (PFPS) it did not do so by altering patella position. Similarly, Gigante et al (2001) in a study using computerised tomography (CT) found that patella lateral position or tilt were not significantly affected by patella taping.

Several studies have concluded that ankle taping to prevent ankle inversion injuries does effectively limit joint range of motion (ROM). Examples include: Cordova et al (2000) who concluded that at least for a period of time tape limits dorsiflexion ROM; Fumich et al (1981) who reported that it limits inversion, eversion, plantarflexion and dorsiflexion; and Gross et al (1994) who found that tape limits inversion and eversion. In an often cited study Vaes et al (1985) conducted a radiological study on the influence of ankle bandaging and taping on talar tilt before and after exercise and found that tape resulted in a significant reduction of tibiotalar instability that persisted even after a 30-minute exercise program.

The low dye foot anti-pronation taping technique has also been found to have immediate effects on foot biomechanics. Harradine et al (2001) found that low dye taping immediately changed calcaneal position in standing but this effect was lost after exercise. Similarly, Constantinou et al (2000) conducted a 3D analysis of the effects of an augmented low dye taping on vertical navicular height and found that the tape did initially increase vertical navicular height, but this effect was reduced after 20 minutes of running. A similar conclusion was made by Vicenzino et al (2005) who found that low dye taping produced a significant immediate increase in medial longitudinal arch (MLA) height in patients who exhibited a navicular drop of more than 10 mm.

While discussing the use of tape to modify the mechanics of the body it is appropriate to make brief mention of the mechanical characteristics of strapping tape. While the tape usually used in musculoskeletal treatments is usually described as 'rigid' and 'adhesive' the rigidity and adhesion of tape alters with time. Several studies have examined the degree and duration of mechanical support provided by tape, especially during dynamic movements such as in sport and exercise and various authors have concluded that mechanical support is reduced over time. For example, Ator et al (1991) found that taping to support the medial longitudinal arch of the foot was significantly diminished after 10 minutes of jogging. It is important for therapists to be aware that there is considerable variation in the quality and performance of different brands and types of tape, and also that the performance can vary under different conditions. Some research relating to the characteristics of strapping tape have been undertaken and some of the findings are discussed in the section 'characteristics of tape and adhesives', Chapter 3, page 21. However, it certainly appears that this is an area that in particular requires more research.

Another approach to the use of tape as a means to changing joint mechanics is as an adjunct to the mobilisation with movement (MWM) techniques described by Mulligan (1999). In this approach it is postulated that tape can be used to maintain the joint position once pain relief has been achieved with a mobilising technique. Papers that have studied this approach include O'Brien and Vicenzino (1998) who used rigid tape to maintain a sustained posterior glide of the fibula on patients with acute ankle sprains and found rapid relief of pain occurred, as well as a rapid increase in the range of inversion and dorsiflexion. In a prospective study on fibular repositioning tape as described by Mulligan, it was found by Moiler et al (2006) that the odds ratio of sustaining an ankle injury in male basketball players was significantly less than for the control group. Other studies that have concluded that Mulligan's MWM techniques combined with tape produced positive outcomes include: Vicenzino and Wright (1995) who reported a case study of a patient with lateral epicondylalgia; Hetherington (1996) with a case study on ankle sprains (cited by Vicenzino et al [2007b]); O'Brien and Vicenzino (1998) with a single case study on an ankle sprain; and Horton (2002) with a case study on a locked thoracic zygoapophyseal joint (cited by Vicenzino et al [2007b]).

Neuromuscular effects: muscle facilitation and/or inhibition

Another proposed use of tape in musculoskeletal practice is to promote normal muscle activation patterns, either by facilitating underactive muscles, or by inhibiting overactive muscles. However, studies into whether tape can successfully and consistently be used to either facilitate or inhibit muscle activity have produced varied results. Also, there is a lack of agreement regarding the mechanism by which tape can cause either facilitation or inhibition of muscle activity, though Vicenzino (2003) concluded that while the research findings so far were inconclusive they do suggest that changes in muscle activity are associated with sensory or mechanical effects produced by the tape.

From an analysis of several studies possible reasons for the variability of the findings could include that the actual taping techniques examined in different studies have varied, or that some studies examined symptomatic subjects while others examined the effects on subjects without symptoms, and also that in some studies statistical power was low due to low numbers of subjects examined in some of the studies and therefore adversely impact the conclusions drawn.

A common assumption or proposed theoretical basis to explain the use of tape to facilitate or inhibit muscle activity is that tape applied across the line of the muscle fibres will inhibit muscle activity, while tape applied in line with muscle fibres will facilitate their action. Across fibre taping to inhibit muscle activity is also often combined with compression, tractioning or gathering of the overlying soft tissues. While this proposition has not been examined in detail possible mechanisms for this effect include the suggestion by Parkhurst and Burnett (1994) that bunching muscle fibres may interfere with actin/myosin cross bridging and therefore reduce muscle function. Following these principles, taping designed to facilitate muscle activity is usually laid onto the skin without soft tissue manipulation or pressure.

A number of research studies have concluded that taping techniques can inhibit muscle activity. Alexander et al (2003) examined the proposition made by Morrissey (2000) that tape applied to the skin over the upper trapezius muscle would increase activity of this muscle as a result of the stimulation of subcutaneous mechanoreceptors. However, these authors found that in fact the opposite occurred and that the amplitude of the upper trapezius H reflex, as evoked by an electrical stimulus, was reduced by underwrap tape applied to the skin over the direction of the muscle fibres, and further reduced when rigid tape was applied under tension to healthy subjects. Morin et al (1997) examined upper, middle and lower trapezius electromyography (EMG) activity in 10 healthy subjects during a scapular stabilisation task and found that tape applied across the upper trapezius resulted in a statistically significant reduction in upper trapezius activity and a commensurate increase in middle and lower trapezius activity. Selkowitz et al (2007) also measured EMG activity but this was in a group of 21 subjects with shoulder pain due to suspected shoulder impingement. They found that upper trapezius activity with tape was significantly lower than without tape during two movement tasks.

Alexander et al (2008) similarly studied the effect of tape on both the medial and the lateral heads of gastrocnemius and found that tape aligned along the direction of the muscle fibres of medial gastrocnemius reduced electrical excitability in both muscles, while tape aligned across the fibres had no effect.

However, the subjects in this study were all free from joint or muscle pain, or suffering from any rheumatological or neurological conditions.

Franettovich et al (2007a) compared foot arch height and EMG activity of six lower leg muscles during walking in 12 asymptomatic subjects before and after walking both un-taped and also with an augmented low dye taping (described on page 185) applied. In this study a concurrent increase in foot arch height and a significant reduction in peak muscle activity in the tibialis posterior, soleus and tibialis anterior muscles were recorded for the subjects while taped.

In contrast to the studies cited above, some researchers have reported that tape neither increases nor decreases muscle activity. Cools et al (2002) recorded surface EMG from the upper trapezius, middle trapezius, lower trapezius and serratus anterior of 20 healthy subjects during full range shoulder abduction and forward flexion and found no significant difference between un-taped subjects and subjects with a strip of tape applied over the muscle belly of upper trapezius and extending inferiorly across the middle and lower trapezius towards the thoracic spine. Similarly in a knee study Cowan et al (2006) found that patella taping did not change the amplitude of EMG in vastus medialis obliquus (VMO) or vastus lateralis (VL) in subjects with patellofemoral pain or control subjects.

One study that did find that tape may increase muscle activity was conducted by Macgregor et al (2005) who found that stretching of the skin over the patella via taping did increase the activity of VMO as measured by EMG, possibly by stimulation of cutaneous afferent receptors in the overlying skin. They further found that lateral stretching of the skin produced a greater increase in amplitude than medial stretching, and that superior stretch produced no increase in VMO activity. This result appears broadly consistent with the findings of Ryan and Rowe (2006)

who found a greater increase in the VMO to VL ratio with lateral taping of the patella, compared to medial taping.

Another study that also reported an increase in muscle activity as measured by EMG, however with a possibly deleterious result, was undertaken by Ackermann et al (2002) who examined the effects of scapula taping on professional violinists while playing. In this study upper trapezius activity increased 49% overall and up to 60% in musical pieces rated as the most physically demanding. At the same time the playing performances of the musicians playing while taped was rated lower by raters who were blinded to the taped or un-taped conditions of the players. Furthermore, the violinists rated their personal confidence and comfort as lower when taped.

Other studies have concentrated on the effect of tape on the timing of the onset of muscle contraction. Cowan et al (2002b) found that therapeutic patella tape altered the timing of onset of VMO and VL in a stair-stepping task in subjects with patellofemoral pain, while the same study and also one by Bennell et al (2006) found that neither therapeutic nor control tape had any effect on VMO to VL onset timing difference in asymptomatic subjects. However, McCarthy Persson et al (2009) found that inhibitory taping applied to the lateral thigh did change VL timing in asymptomatic subjects. Herrington and Payton (1997) found that, while pain decreased with taping, a concurrent increase in VMO EMG activity was not statistically significant.

McCarthy Persson et al (2007) conducted a study to examine if the variables of skin displacement and skin pressure were repeatable in a technique designed to inhibit activity of VL, arguing that 'studies of the effects of taping are of little consequence if the taping procedure itself cannot be replicated'. Based on their examination of these variables they concluded that taping designed to inhibit VL produced a reproducible effect for skin displacement, but not for skin pressure. However, all procedures and measures were conducted by the same researcher which weakens the generalisability of these conclusions. Once again, it is our opinion that more research into the reproducibility and accuracy of the application of taping techniques, as well as any effects associated with the skill level and experience of the operator, appear to be warranted.

PROPRIOCEPTION ENHANCEMENT

Another proposed benefit of taping by authors such as Myburgh et al (1984) and Karlsson and Andreasson (1992) is that it can enhance proprioceptive ability, thereby stimulating enhanced muscular control around the targeted area. Many proponents of this approach as a factor in injury prevention argue that tactile stimulation of the skin provided by the tape can stimulate cutaneous nerve receptors, or muscle or joint mechanoreceptors, which in turn can result in earlier and/or enhanced activation of the protective muscle reflex arc (Heit et al 1996). However, the findings of different studies are inconsistent with regard to whether tape has an effect on proprioception.

Studies that claim evidence of proprioceptive enhancement that can be attributed to tape include Heit et al (1996) who measured the ability of 26 subjects to accurately reproduce ankle joint angles while either taped with a standardised anti-inversion taping of anchors, 4 stirrups, horseshoe strips and heel locks, compared to being braced with a Swede-O-Universal ankle support, or with no external support. They concluded that tape significantly increased the subject's joint position sense in both plantar flexion and inversion compared to either bracing or no support.

Lohrer et al (1999) described a 'proprioceptive amplification ratio' based on reflex EMG traces and maximum inversion amplitude in 40 subjects exposed to an inversion injury simulation. Adhesive tape was also applied which produced a reported immediate increase in ankle stability, which, although decreased by exercise performed while the tape was in situ, increased the proprioceptive amplification ratio. However, whether an increase in ankle stability and true proprioceptive enhancement are comparable is of course debatable. Karlsson and Andreasson (1992) however reported that reaction time of the peroneal muscles as measured by EMG was significantly reduced in 20 mechanically unstable ankles with tape applied, possibly as an effect of cutaneous stimulation by the tractioning force of tape on the skin. Similarly, Gilleard et al (1998) reported that patella taping changed the timing of VL and VM onset in patients with patella femoral pain, with earlier activation of vastus medialis occurring in both a step-down and step-up task. Robbins et al (1995) found that foot position error was 107.5% poorer with athletic footwear than barefoot, but with ankle taping foot position error was 58.1% worse than barefoot. They also found that after exercise foot position error was 2.5% when taped compared to 35.5% worse when un-taped and concluded that ankle taping partly corrects the negative effect on proprioception of athletic footwear and exercise.

One study that indicates tape does increase joint position awareness, but not under all conditions, was conducted by Simoneau et al (1997). They examined whether tape increases proprioception by increasing stimulation of mechanoreceptors in the skin. In this study ankle joint position perception and ankle joint movement perception was measured in 20 healthy male subjects, with and without a single 12.7 cm strip of tape applied vertically over the anterior ankle, and another posteriorly over the Achilles tendon and the calcaneum. They found that taping significantly improved perception of ankle joint position in non-weight bearing, but not while weight bearing. The authors reasoned that the tape could help in proper positioning of the ankle immediately prior to impact in running or jumping and that this may be a factor in reducing ankle sprains. There was no significant improvement in joint movement perception between the taped and un-taped groups reported in this study.

Callaghan et al (2002) found no overall between-group differences of patella taping versus no taping on three tests of proprioception in a sample of 52 subjects. However, they did find that based on a within-group analysis subjects rated as having poor proprioceptive ability did exhibit enhanced scores on the proprioceptive tests when taped. These results are similar to those reported by Cameron et al (2008) who found that neoprene shorts enhanced leg proprioception, as measured by leg swing judgment, in Australian football players who were judged to have low neuromuscular control ability, but that the neoprene shorts reduced leg swing judgment in players of high neuromuscular control ability.

Some studies have found that taping has no evidence of effect on proprioception; for example, Allison et al (1999). This study investigated the peroneal reflex response to rapid inversion using a trapdoor with different taping protocols. The dominant leg of 31 healthy subjects was tested in three conditions: no taping; simple prophylactic taping; and circumferential leg taping. A repeated measures Analysis of Variance (ANOVA) revealed no statistically significant effect across conditions or trials. According to these authors the results suggest that neurophysiological responses to sudden inversion are not altered by mechanical or sensory input from taping in normal subjects. Hinman et al (2004) found that patella taping had no effect on sensorimotor function in the short or medium term on people with knee joint osteoarthritis.

Broglio et al (2009) concluded that ankle taping and bracing devices actually had a negative effect on postural control as measured on the balance error scoring system (BESS), which they hypothesised as being due to decreased ankle mobility. Unfortunately the method of ankle taping used in the study was not described. Refshauge et al (2009) similarly concluded that tape had a negative effect on the ability of subjects with recurrent ankle sprains to detect ankle movements when a standard anti-inversion ankle taping consisting of stirrups, figure 6s and heel locks was applied.

With the inconsistent findings the question remains as to whether tape has a definite effect on enhancement of proprioception, and also on muscle facilitation and inhibition generally, or if the benefits are limited to subjects with reduced or altered function due to pain or pathology.

DELOADING AND/OR UNLOADING TECHNIQUES

Some techniques used by therapists are based on the proposition that tape can be used to reduce strain on soft tissues, usually by an application of tape that approximates muscle tissue around the site of pain or injury. These techniques are usually described as either tissue deloading or sometimes unloading techniques.

Based on the principle of deloading a number of techniques have been developed for several body regions, some of which are presented in this book. A number of these techniques are described as box taping or diamond taping techniques as the tape is applied end to end, surrounding and gathering the tissues towards the painful area for the purpose of unloading pain-producing tissues.

McConnell (2000) proposed that tape could be used to 'unload' painful structures and that with reduced pain a therapist has an opportunity to direct treatment at the underlying cause or causes. The described premise in this article is that tape can be used to shorten and reduce stress on inflamed tissues with the result being decreased pain. In the same paper the author presented three case studies where tape applied with a tractioning force was successfully used as an adjunct to treatment. In another article in 2002 the same author (McConnell 2002) stated that while unloading tape works clinically, research had thus far been unable to determine the exact mechanism. Examination of the literature since 2002 does not seem to alter this view.

O'Leary et al (2002) conducted a study to determine if a deloading taping technique affected the perception of pain to applied pressure on the spinous processes of T7 of a group of asymptomatic subjects. They found no significant change in pressure pain thresholds in this asymptomatic group and recommended further research with symptomatic subjects, speculating further that patients with hyperalgesia may show a greater response to taping.

Studies that have investigated the use of deloading tape in symptomatic subjects though limited in number are so far encouraging as to its effect. For example, Vicenzino et al (2003) described a diamond taping technique for reducing pain due to lateral epicondylagia as an adjunct to exercise. This technique also involved four strips of tape applied to the skin around the painful area while a tractioning force was applied to gather the tissues. The authors reported that this technique improved pain-free grip strength both immediately and up to 30 minutes after application, while the placebo and sham treatment and control groups demonstrated little effect.

Another proposed effect for taping in the deloading group is that it displaces subcutaneous tissues, including the fascia. Alexander (2007) reported that real time ultrasound demonstrated that tape using a similar gathering technique directed transversely to the thoraco-lumbar fascia displaced the transversus abdominis and its fascia in the direction of the tape, and similarly that tape applied longitudinally to the quadriceps also resulted in longitudinal displacement of subcutaneous

tissues. However, the number of subjects these conclusions were based on was not stated in this report and no follow-up randomised controlled clinical trials (RCTs) or similar high-level evidence have been published to date.

Another group of studies that potentially could be considered as evidence for the use of tape to unload painful tissues are those related to the use of tape as an adjunct to the Mulligan MWM techniques, already examined in the section on the mechanical effects of tape. As is the case for many conditions, a clear distinction between how bodily systems are primarily modified by the described treatments is at best difficult, and more likely than not in some cases represent an oversimplification of what are complex, interrelated processes.

PSYCHOLOGICAL EFFECTS

Another possible effect of taping is psychological impact. While mentioned as a possible effect by several authors very few articles were found that directly investigated the psychological effects of tape on subjects. Hunt and Short (2006) interviewed 11 athletes who routinely taped their ankles either post injury or for injury prevention and concluded that taping resulted in feelings of increased confidence in athletes who had not sustained an injury. In athletes who were using ankle tape as a result of an injury, and those who had not been injured, tape resulted in feelings of increased strength and decreased anxiety about sustaining an injury or re-injury. Conversely though, Ackermann et al (2002) studied the effect of a taping technique designed to promote optimal scapula positioning and support in professional violinists, however, the musicians reported a reduction in confidence and comfort. At the same time the application of tape was rated by other listeners as having a negative effect on playing performance.

THE EFFECTS OF TAPE ON OEDEMA

Tape has been suggested as a method to reduce oedema, primarily through its compressive effect and especially post injury. Capasso et al (1989) measured the pressure under three different types of adhesive tapes and two non-adhesive bandages applied to the ankle and concluded that adhesive bandages were more effective than non-adhesive bandages in their compressive ability on the ankle to prevent swelling, especially with prolonged application.

Shim et al (2003) conducted a study to investigate whether elastic adhesive tape would increase lymphatic flow in the hind legs of rabbits, on the basis that 'any method that deforms the skin of the extremities may increase lymphatic flow'. Based on their study, in which lymphatic flow was calculated both at rest and during passive exercise from the hind legs of 22 rabbits, they concluded that:

○ tape plus passive exercise significantly increased lymph flow rate
○ tape without exercise had no effect on lymph flow
○ if the area of the tape was increased lymph flow rates increased linearly
○ tape on the anterior ankle caused greater deformation than on the dorsum of the foot, and this was associated with a tendency to increase lymph flow rate more.

The authors concluded that elastic adhesive tape combined with passive exercise increased lymph flow rate by deforming the skin and suggested that this method could be used in the treatment of lymphatic oedema. This was the only study identified that directly examined the effects of tape on lymphatic flow.

KINETIC TYPE TAPING

Kinetic type taping is an approach to taping that has evolved relatively recently, and utilises a specific type of brand-marked elastic tape that is designed to mimic the qualities of human skin and is applied in specific ways. The proposed multiple benefits of kinetic type taping techniques include provision of positional stimulus through the skin, fascial alignment, sensory stimulation to assist or limit motion, unloading of painful or inflamed soft tissues, and oedema removal through enhanced lymphatic drainage (Thelen et al 2008). The same authors also conducted a well-designed randomised, double-blinded clinical trial on the effects of Kinesio® taping on subjects with shoulder pain and found that the group who received Kinesio® taping had a significant immediate improvement in pain-free shoulder abduction, although by day 3 post treatment there were no differences between the two groups, possibly indicating that its benefit may be limited to providing pain reduction immediately post treatment. At the time of writing other high quality published studies examining the benefits of Kinesio® taping are limited, however Fu et al (2008) conducted a study on the effects of Kinesio® taping on quadriceps and hamstring strength before, immediately after application, and 12 hours post application of Kinesio® taping and found no significant difference between the three conditions. In contrast with this study Slupik et al (2007) found that Kinesio® tape applied to the quadriceps increased peak torque that persisted even after the tape was removed.

More research into this system of taping is necessary before any conclusions regarding its benefit or superiority over other approaches to taping can be made. It is not the aim of this edition to describe any techniques utilising this type of elastic tape.

CHARACTERISTICS OF TAPE AND ADHESIVES

A small number of studies have examined different types and characteristics of tape, including the types of fabric and adhesives, as well as the effects of the tape on the skin interface. The results of these studies may influence a therapist's choice of tape depending on the effects sought.

Several studies have identified that tape used for limiting ankle ROM loses its effectiveness after approximately 20 minutes of exercise; for example, Fumich et al (1981), Greene and Hillman (1990), Laughman et al (1980) and Myburgh et al (1984). This loss of resistive force could be related to fatigue or stretching of the tape material, reduction in the adhesive's effectiveness, changes in the skin/tape interface, or a combination of these factors.

A comparison of the breaking strain and fatigue under load characteristics of two types of rigid tape, Zonas and Leukotape, and an elastic adhesive tape, Jaylastic, was conducted by Bragg et al (2002). They found that after 20 minutes of a force applied cyclically to the different tapes that 21% (Zonas), 29% (Leukotape) and 57% (Jaylastic) of the mechanical support of the tape was lost. Leukotape had a greater breaking strain than Zonas and both rigid tapes had significantly greater breaking strengths than the elastic tape. Microscopic examination of the microstructure of the tape determined that Zonas and Leukotape had approximately the same number of fibres per width in the direction of the applied load, however, Leukotape also has secondary fibres orientated at approximately 45 degrees to the direction of loading which also contribute a resultant resistance component.

Beringer (2008) compared the adhesiveness of four different brands of adhesive tapes under three different skin conditions — wet, dry or with prior application of Friars' Balsam (compound benzoin tincture). Using a strain gauge to measure the force required to detach tape he determined that Leukoplast zinc oxide was more adhesive than Sleek, Mefix and Elastoplast, in that order. Under wet conditions the adhesiveness of Leukoplast and Sleek was unchanged, whereas Elastoplast and Mefix were less adhesive. The application of Friars' Balsam significantly increased adhesiveness of Elastoplast and Sleek.

Other studies that have investigated the effect of different tape adhesives and the effect on skin include Tokumura et al (2006) who found that the dermal peeling force required to remove tape and the resultant stripping of corneocytes from the skin is lower with tapes that are less permeable to water, possibly because of greater fluid accumulation below the tape. They also found that there were differences between different body regions of dermal peeling for permeable tape, but little difference for impermeable tape. In a separate study Tokumura et al (2007) determined that softer tape adhesives were associated with less pain and less skin trauma when tape was removed.

Karwoski and Plaut (2004) examined the ideal peeling angle to reduce pain and skin trauma related to the removal of adhesive tape and found that the peel force tended to be at a minimum with a peel angle of 150 degrees. Peel force tended to increase with repeated peeling from the same skin test site. This may be related to the accumulation of adhesive material that penetrates into the sulci cutis (skin furrows) as identified by Tokumura et al (2007). Karwoski and Plaut (2004) also found that increased peel rate resulted in a tendency towards increased peel force, but that this relationship was inconsistent.

Sekar and Srinivas (2008) conducted a small study comparing the effectiveness of different solvents on the removal of retained adherent on the skin material from Micropore tape. Acetone and ether were found to be the most effective, followed by spirit, and soap combined with water was the least effective. Skin cleaned with spirit and soap water still demonstrated persistent adherent material even after 48 hours post removal.

SIDE-EFFECTS OF TAPE

Given the frequent anecdotal and also clinical observation of the association between the use of tape and skin irritation surprisingly few studies were found that investigated this connection. This was also the conclusion of Wildman et al (2008) who commented that in the literature there are few reports describing a link between proven allergic contact dermatitis (ACD) and the use of medical adhesive bandages and tapes. According to 3M Health Care (2005) skin reactions from tape that are observed clinically are most commonly related to mechanical trauma to the skin and result in injuries such as skin stripping and tension blisters, and that ACD, irritant contact dermatitis (ICD), folliculitis and skin maceration related to the use of tape are rare. From the available literature this contention appears reasonably well supported.

The proposition that reactions from tape are likely to be as a result of mechanically induced trauma would appear to be supported by the study of Tokumura et al (2005) who examined the effect of repetitive application and removal of two types of adhesive tape with different strength adhesives in a small trial of 6 subjects. They found skin irritation increased with repeated applications and removal, as measured by the amount of stripped corneocytes from the skin, which was in turn associated with greater skin furrowing and increased trans-epidermal water loss. These measures were more pronounced with the stronger adhesive.

Another study that indicates that skin reactions vary depending on the type of tape used was conducted by Koval et al (2003). In a trial of 99 patients who underwent hip surgery they contrasted the use of perforated cloth tape versus non-stretch silk tape applied over the dressing. Of the patients who had the silk tape, 41% developed blisters in the area the tape was applied; 10% of the patients who had the perforated cloth tape developed blisters. They found no association between the development of blisters and age, gender, co-morbidities, smoking, nutrition or surgical procedure.

Wildman et al (2008) conducted a trial of allergy patch tests with 26 patients who had been identified as having ACD associated with tape and bandage adhesives. None of the patients exhibited any positive allergic reactions to 10 different types of tapes and bandages, or 54 other chemicals associated with allergies. However, 8 of the 11 subjects who left a bandage or tape on for 7 days exhibited an irritant reaction. The authors concluded that these reactions were more likely associated with ICD, rather than ACD.

Another study that concluded tape was not causative of skin reactions was conducted by Bartlett et al (1982) who reported an outbreak of boils in an American high school football team. Tape was one of a number of factors associated with the development of boils but its use was not considered to be causal, rather they felt it more likely was reflective of an attempt to protect compromised areas of skin with a high risk of developing boils.

TAPING EFFECTS BY REGION OR CONDITION

The usefulness of taping in the treatment of some particular conditions has been studied quite frequently, while many have received little or no detailed scientific investigation. The following conditions and body regions are ones identified as having a sufficient number of relevant studies to warrant at least a brief summary of the findings.

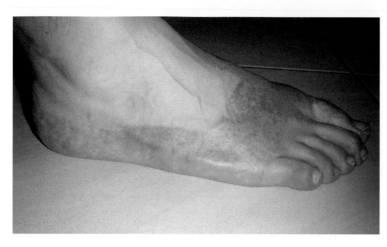

FIGURE 2.2 A PATIENT WITH SKIN IRRITATION FOLLOWING LOW DYE TAPING (THE PATIENT IN THIS CASE HAD THE TAPE IN SITU FOR 2 DAYS)

SCAPULA AND SHOULDER

Scapula taping techniques have been postulated as a beneficial adjunct to treatment for shoulder conditions by several authors. For example, Host (1995) in a single case study design with a patient with chronic shoulder pain described a taping technique to maintain scapula retraction and depression for the purpose of improving poor scapula control as an adjunct to an exercise program.

In a larger study involving 60 subjects diagnosed with signs of subacromial impingement, as well as 60 asymptomatic control subjects, Lewis et al (2005) found that scapular taping effectively changed posture and that this change in posture was associated with increased shoulder forward flexion and also abduction in the scapula plane in the subjects with shoulder pain. They also found that pain-free ROM was increased with the tape, though

pain intensity at the onset of pain was not significantly altered.

Using a technique somewhat similar to that described by Host, but applied bilaterally and with single strips of tape, Greig et al (2008) found definite evidence of a reduced angle of kyphosis that could be attributed to tape in female subjects with osteoporotic fractures. They also found, however, that the taped test condition was not associated with any change in EMG activity and concluded that further research to determine the underlying causes for the changes to the angle of kyphosis is necessary.

Selkowitz et al (2007) measured EMG activity in 21 subjects with shoulder pain due to suspected shoulder impingement and found that scapular taping produced a small but significant reduction in upper trapezius activity in a functional overhead reaching task that primarily involved forward flexion, and also that taping reduced upper trapezius activity during abduction in the plane of the scapula. They also found that lower trapezius activity was increased in the overhead reaching task, but was not altered in the abduction test. Cools et al (2002), however, performed a similar study in 20 healthy subjects with a similar taping technique applied to the scapula and did not find any evidence of any changes in muscle activation or proprioception. Once again, as discussed in the section on neuromuscular effects of tape, the question remains as to whether tape facilitates muscle activity generally, or whether the facilitatory effect is only present in subjects with reduced muscle activity due to pain or pathology, or some other combination of factors.

Not including taping techniques directed at improving scapula position or stability such as those described above, several shoulder taping techniques directed at improving conditions associated with the glenohumeral and acromioclavicular joint, including rotator cuff pathology, have been proposed. Many of these are based on a well-reasoned theoretical basis; however, not many studies relating to the clinical effectiveness of these shoulder taping techniques have been published, especially for techniques directed at the glenohumeral joint. As an example of this approach Kneeshaw (2002) published an article that described a number of shoulder taping techniques where origins were attributed to several different clinicians. Most of the described techniques were accompanied with a proposed rationale but no supporting clinical trials.

It was also an interesting finding of our literature review that, despite the fact that shoulder taping has been used commonly in sports as an injury prevention strategy, very few studies were identified that examine its effectiveness in shoulder injury prevention. One recently published study by Bradley et al (2009) examined the use of a particular type of shoulder taping on inferior glenohumeral joint laxity, as well as on joint position sense and also a handball passing task in 33 Australian Football League players. They concluded that tape did not significantly affect any of the three tested parameters and therefore was of no benefit. However, the shoulder taping techniques used in this population are usually designed to reduce anterior glenohumeral laxity rather than inferior laxity as was tested in this study, so whether the conclusion made by the authors that taping is of no benefit can be generalised in such a way is debatable.

In a non-sporting population a study that did demonstrate some evidence of effect for prevention of shoulder symptoms was undertaken by Griffin and Bernhardt (2006) who conducted a prospective randomised controlled trial (RCT) in 36 stroke patients. They found that therapeutic shoulder taping reduced the likelihood of high-risk patients developing hemiplegic shoulder pain compared to patients who received a placebo taping, or patients who received no taping.

With regard to the use of taping for the treatment of symptoms related to acromioclavicular (AC) joint separation, two studies were identified. The first study was a single case study by Stoddard and Johnson (2000) that used taping to promote stability and increased pain free ROM as an adjunct to treatment in a patient with a partial AC joint separation. The second study was a paper by Shamus and Shamus (1997) that described a taping technique that was used in two patients both diagnosed with Grade III AC joint injuries. In this study the authors reported that both patients attributed substantial pain relief to the support provided by the taping. However, the conclusions of this paper were compromised not only by the small sample size and lack of a control group, but also by the fact that the two patients were also concurrently receiving other physical therapy treatment, including ice and exercises.

ELBOW LATERAL EPICONDYLALGIA

Many patients with pain and weakness due to lateral epicondylalgia use counterforce braces that compress the forearm muscles with the goal of changing the functional mechanical origin of the extensor muscles. While most studies relating to the use of counterforce techniques for lateral epicondylalgia specifically have examined pre-made braces, taping can be used to replicate the effects of a counterforce brace, and a technique for this is included on page 76.

Clinically, many patients ascribe significant pain relief to counterforce bracing or taping; a view supported by Forbes and Hopper (1990). However, in their study of 19 tennis players with elbow pain they found that counterforce braces had no significant effect on grip strength. Anderson and Rutt (1992) similarly found no evidence that counterforce braces affected forearm muscle strength of normal subjects during isokinetic dynamometer testing. Chan and Ng (2003) found that counterforce braces have no effect on wrist extensor muscle performance in normal subjects, but that they do increase the pain threshold when wrist extensors were passively stretched to the onset of pain. A similar conclusion was reported by the same authors from another published study (Ng & Chan 2004).

However, tape has been demonstrated to be effective in the treatment of lateral epicondylalgia with a deloading technique. Based on a study with 16 patients with chronic lateral epicondylalgia, Vicenzino et al (2003) found that a diamond-shaped deloading technique (as described on page 74) significantly increased pain-free grip strength.

PATELLOFEMORAL PAIN

A large number of the studies relevant to the use of tape for the treatment of musculoskeletal conditions specifically relate to patellofemoral pain syndrome (PFPS). Several studies reported that medial patella taping reduced PFPS pain, including Bockrath et al (1993), Cushnaghan et al (1994), Somes et al (1997), Herrington and Payton (1997), Powers et al (1997), Salsich et al (2002), Wilson et al (2003), and Crossley et al (2009). In some cases the authors specifically reported that the decrease in pain due to patella taping was immediate. In contrast, Kowall et al (1996) and Keet et al (2007) found no statistically significant decrease in pain due to patella taping.

One study that investigated the effect of patella taping on a functional outcome was conducted by Powers et al (1997) who found that taping increased stride length in patients with PFPS pain. This increase was also associated with a 78% reduction in pain as measured by the visual analogue scale (VAS). The authors in this study concluded that the decrease in pain may have been primarily causative of the improvement in function, rather than direct biomechanical changes caused by the tape.

There are other studies that are also inconclusive or contradictory as to whether patella taping achieves its pain producing results at least in part through mechanical re-

alignment of the patella. For example, Gigante et al (2001) conducted a study using computerised tomography (CT) that concluded that patella taping did not significantly change patella orientation with regard to lateral position or tilt, while Pfeiffer et al (2004) studied medial glide patella taping at four angles with magnetic resonance imaging (MRI) and found that tape resulted in significant medial displacement, although this alteration was not maintained after exercise. Worrell et al (1998) also examined the effect of taping and bracing with MRI and concluded that both did increase medial patella displacement, though only at 10 degrees of knee flexion.

Several studies indicated that patella taping has an effect on EMG activity or the timing of the onset of muscle activation, though the findings are inconsistent or inconclusive; for example, Cowan et al (2002a), Cowan et al (2006). This view is supported by Fagan and Delahunt (2008) who concluded that more studies are needed to establish the true efficacy of patella taping on VMO and VL activation patterns. The effect of tape on muscle facilitation is covered in more detail in the earlier section on muscle facilitation and inhibition on page 15.

In conclusion, as far as the use of tape for PFPS is concerned, with the large number of papers relating to the use of patella taping and the inconsistent results it is difficult to surmise conclusively the benefits or otherwise of taping from any of the studies in isolation. Overington et al (2006) did conduct a critical appraisal of 21 studies related to the use of patella taping for patellofemoral pain that were deemed of sufficiently high quality for inclusion in their review based on the PEDro rating scale. They concluded that patella taping does reduce pain in the short term, does alter EMG characteristics and may be useful in the long-term management of patellofemoral pain. Somewhat similarly, Aminaka and Gribble (2005) conducted a systematic review on the use of taping for PFPS and concluded that taping does appear to reduce pain and improve function but that evidence was limited and further research was indicated.

ANKLE SPRAIN PREVENTION

Many of the studies regarding the use of tape for the ankle relate to its role in injury prevention, or re-injury prevention, especially during sport. According to Arnold and Docherty (2004) several studies and reviews support the view that taping does reduce the likelihood of ankle sprain; however, as to whether the main reason for the reduction is mechanical restriction of movement, enhancement of proprioception or balance (Barkoukis et al 2002; Bennell & Goldie 1994), preferential joint positioning while landing from a step or a jump, increased strength of muscle contraction (Ashton-Miller et al 1996), or a combination of any or all of these is not clear.

Due to the large number of studies published regarding ankle sprains only a selection of the key findings and reviews have been presented here. A number of authors have conducted comprehensive reviews on the role and effectiveness of taping for ankle injury prevention, including Olmstead et al (2004) who conducted a review of articles relating to taping for ankle injury prevention that contained sufficient data to conduct a numbers needed to treat (NNT) analysis. From their analysis of the papers identified in their review they calculated that:

○ from a study of basketball players the prevention of one ankle sprain required the taping of 26 players who had a history of a previous ankle sprain, and 143 players who had not had a previous injury
○ from a second study of basketball players the NNT was 18 for those with a previous injury and 39 with no previous history
○

○ from a study of soccer players the NNT for players with a history of injury was 5, compared to 57 for those without a previous injury.

Not surprisingly from these results they concluded that the protective effects are greater for athletes with a previous history of ankle sprains. The same authors also performed a cost benefit analysis using this NNT basis and calculated that ankle taping was approximately three times more expensive than bracing. Other studies that also have concluded that taping or bracing confers a protective effect include Firer (1990), Gray (1991) and Mickel et al (2006). Some studies have further identified that tape tends to lose some of its mechanical resistance to inversion with exercise; for example, Gross et al (1991) and Myburgh et al (1984).

The protective effects conferred by taping may also come at a cost in performance. For example, Burks et al (1991) found that ankle taping resulted in a significant decrease in athletic performance measures such as vertical jump height, shuttle run and sprint time. Similarly Mackean et al (1995) found tape and bracing reduced vertical jump height and increased oxygen consumption. Providing a slightly different perspective was Thacker et al (1999) who conducted a review of 113 studies reporting the risk of ankle sprains in sports and concluded that most studies indicated that taping or bracing does not reduce performance, however only 20 of the 113 studies measured the effects of taping or bracing on running, jumping or agility skills such as cutting and figure 8 running.

PLANTAR FASCIITIS

A number of studies have found that taping, especially the low dye or augmented low dye technique to increase medial longitudinal arch (MLA) height and reduce pronation, can have a positive benefit in the treatment of plantar fasciitis, presumably through reduction of tensile stress at the attachment of the fascia to the calcaneum. Studies that have concluded that taping decreases pain from plantar fasciitis, and sometimes other symptoms such as stiffness, include Osborne et al (2006), Hyland et al (2006), Jamali et al (2004) and Meyer et al (2002). Studies that have demonstrated that taping does positively affect parameters such as increased MLA height include Vicenzino et al (2000), Vicenzino et al (2005) and Radford et al (2006); decreased plantar foot pressures O'Sullivan et al (2008) and Vicenzino et al (2007a).

In addition, Bartold et al (2009) conducted a study on plantar fascia taping on cadaveric feet utilising in-dwelling strain gauges and found that taping directly reduces the strain within the plantar fascia. Franettovich et al (2008) found that anti-pronation taping reduced EMG activity of tibialis posterior, tibialis anterior and peroneus longus in subjects with low MLA and in another paper that the changes in muscle activation patterns were maintained even after the taping was removed (Franettovich et al 2007b).

Taken together there is considerable evidence for the effectiveness of taping as a treatment for plantar fasciitis both in the acute phase, and also in ongoing management.

SUMMARY

There is considerable evidence that tape is an effective adjunct to treatment in the management of a number of musculoskeletal conditions. However, there are also a number of studies that question the validity of taping, or the underlying assumptions as to its effects. As for all clinical treatments the authors recommend that taping techniques are always used in conjunction with relevant outcome measures to assist in the analysis of change in the condition of each individual patient. Valid outcome measures will assist therapists in determining if a taping technique appears to be contributing to improved outcomes or, in lieu of improvement of the patient's condition, whether another approach to treatment should be considered.

REFERENCES

3M Health Care (2005) Reducing the risk of superficial skin damage related to adhesive use. Online. Available: http://multimedia.3m.com/mws/mediawebserver?66666UuZjcFSLXTtMx&_5X&EEVuQEcuZgVs6EVs6E666666 (accessed 30 September 2009).

Ackermann, B, Adams, R & Marshall, E (2002) The effect of scapula taping on electromyographic activity and musical performance in professional violinists. The Australian Journal of Physiotherapy, 197–203.

Alexander, C M, Mcmullan, M, Harrison, P J (2008) What is the effect of taping along or across a muscle on motoneuron excitability? A study using triceps surae. Manual Therapy, 13(1): 57–62.

Alexander, C M, Stynes, S, Thomas, A, Lewis, J & Harrison, P J (2003) Does tape facilitate or inhibit the lower fibres of trapezius? Manual Therapy, 8(1): 37–41.

Alexander, R (2007) Real Time Ultrasound Investigation. Inaugural Fascia Research Congress, Harvard Medical School, Boston.

Allison, G T, Hopper, D, Martin, L, Tillberg, N & Woodhouse, D (1999) The influence of rigid taping on peroneal latency in normal ankles. Australian Journal of Physiotherapy, 45(3): 195–201.

Aminaka, N & Gribble, P A (2005) A systematic review of the effects of therapeutic taping on patellofemoral pain syndrome (structured abstract). Journal of Athletic Training, 341–51.

Anderson, M A & Rutt, R A (1992) The effects of counterforce bracing on forearm and wrist muscle function. Journal of Orthopaedic & Sports Physical Therapy, 87–91.

Arnold, B L & Docherty, C L (2004) Bracing and rehabilitation — what's new. Clinics in Sports Medicine, 23(1): 83–95.

Ashton-Miller, J A, Ottaviani, R A, Hutchinson, C & Wojtys, E M (1996) What best protects the inverted weight bearing ankle against further inversion? Evertor muscle strength compares favorably with shoe height, athletic tape, and three orthoses. American Journal of Sports Medicine, 24(6): 800–9.

Ator, R, Gunn, K, Mcpoil, T & Knecht, H (1991) The effect of adhesive strapping on medial longitudinal arch support before and after exercise. Journal of Orthopaedic & Sports Physical Therapy, 14(1): 18–23.

Barkoukis, V, Sykaras, E, Costa, F & Tsorbatzoudis, H (2002) Effectiveness of taping and bracing in balance. Perceptual and Motor Skills, 94(2): 566–74.

Bartlett, P C, Martin, R J & Cahill, B R (1982) Furunculosis in a high school football team. The American Journal of Sports Medicine, 10(6): 371–4.

Bartold, S, Clarke, R, Franklyn-Miller, A, Falvey, E, Bryant, A, Briggs, C & McCrory, R (2009) The effect of taping on plantar fascia strain: a cadaveric study. Journal of Science and Medicine in Sport, 12(suppl 1): S74–S75.

Bennell, K, Duncan, M & Cowan, S (2006) Effect of patellar taping on vasti onset timing, knee kinematics, and kinetics in asymptomatic individuals with a delayed onset of vastus medialis oblique. Journal of Orthopaedic Research, 24, 1854–60.

Bennell, K L & Goldie, P A (1994) The differential effects of external ankle support on postural control. Journal of Orthopaedic & Sports Physical Therapy, 20(6): 287–95.

Beringer, R (2008) Study of the adhesiveness of medical tapes when wet, dry or following application of Friars' Balsam. Paediatric Anaesthesia, 18(6): 520–4.

Berkowitz, M & Bottoni, C R (2006) Taping and bracing contest ankle sprain. Biomechanics Archives: July 2006. Online. Available: http://www.biomech.com/full_article/?ArticleID=457&month=07&year=2006 (accessed 19 September 2009).

Bockrath, K, Wooden, C, Worrell, T, Ingersoll, C & Farr, J (1993) Effects of patella taping on patella position and perceived pain. Medicine & Science in Sports & Exercise, 25(9): 989–92.

Bradley, C B, Fischer, D, Murrell, G (2009) The effect of taping on the shoulders of AFL football players. British Journal of Sports Medicine, 43:735–8 (published online first: 16 July 2009 doi:10.1136/bjsm.2008.049858).

Bragg, R W, MacMahon, J M, Overom, E K, Yerby, S A, Matheson, G O, Carter, D R & Andriacchi, T P (2002) Failure and fatigue characteristics of adhesive athletic tape. Medicine & Science in Sports & Exercise, 34(3): 403–10.

Broglio, S, Monk, A, Sopiarz, K & Cooper, E (2009) The influence of ankle support on postural control. Journal of Science & Medicine in Sport, 12(3): 388–92.

Burks, R T, Bean, B G, Marcus, R & Barker, H B (1991) Analysis of athletic performance with prophylactic ankle devices. The American Journal of Sports Medicine, 19(2): 104–106.

Callaghan, M J, Selfe, J, Bagley, P J, Oldham, J A (2002) The effects of patellar taping on knee joint proprioception. Journal of Athletic Training, 37(1): 19–24.

Cameron, M L, Adams, R D et al (2008) The effect of neoprene shorts on leg proprioception in Australian football players. Journal of Science and Medicine in Sport, 11(3): 345–52.

Capasso, G, Maffulli, N, Testa, V (1989) Ankle taping: support given by different materials. British Journal of Sports Medicine, 23(4): 239–40.

Chan, H L, Ng, G Y (2003) Effect of counterforce forearm bracing on wrist extensor muscles performance. American Journal of Physical Medicine, Rehabilitation, 290–5.

Constantinou, M, Neal, R, Van Rabenau, F, Watson, K, Vicenzino, B (2000) A 3D kinematic analysis of the effects of anti-pronation taping on the foot: a pilot study. International Congress on Sport Science, Sports Medicine and Physical Education, Brisbane.

Cools, A M, Witvrouw, E E, Danneels, L A, Cambier, D C (2002) Does taping influence electromyographic muscle activity in the scapular rotators in healthy shoulders? Manual Therapy, 7(3): 154–62.

Cordova, M L, Ingersoll, C D, Leblanc, M J (2000) Influence of ankle support on joint range of motion before and after exercise: a meta-analysis. Journal of Orthopaedic, Sports Physical Therapy, 30(4): 170–7.

Cowan, S, Bennell, K, Crossley, K, Hodges, P W, McConnell, J (2002a) Physical therapy alters recruitment of the vasti in patellofemoral pain syndrome. Medicine, Science in Sports, Exercise, 34(12): 1879–85.

Cowan, S M, Bennell, K L, Hodges, P W, Cowan, S M, Bennell, K L, Hodges, P W (2002b) Therapeutic patellar taping changes the timing of vasti muscle activation in people with patellofemoral pain syndrome. Clinical Journal of Sport Medicine, 12(6): 339–47.

Cowan, S M, Hodges, P W, Crossley, K M, Bennell, K L (2006) Patellar taping does not change the amplitude of electromyographic activity of the vasti in a stair stepping task. British Journal of Sports Medicine, 40(1) 30–34.

Crossley, K, Marino, G, Macilquham, M, Schache, A, Hinman, R (2009) The effect of patellar tape on patellar malalignment associated with patellofemoral osteoarthritis. Journal of Science and Medicine in Sport, 12(Suppl 1): S68.

Cushnaghan, J, Mccarthy, R, Dieppe, P (1994) The effect of taping the patella on pain in the osteoarthritic patient. British Medical Journal, 308(308): 753–5.

Fagan, V, Delahunt, E (2008) Patellofemoral pain syndrome: a review on the associated neuromuscular deficits and current treatment options. British Journal of Sports Medicine, 42(10): 789–95.

Firer, P (1990) Effectiveness of taping for the prevention of ankle ligament sprains. British Journal of Sports Medicine, 24(1): 47–50.

Forbes A, Hopper, D (1990) The effect of counterforce bracing on grip strength in tennis players with painful elbows. Australian Journal of Physiotherapy, 259–65.

Franettovich, M, Chapman, A, Blanch, P, Vicenzino, B (2007a) Augmented low dye tape induced changes in muscle activation are maintained whilst mechanical effects are reduced with activity. Journal of Science and Medicine in Sport, 10(suppl 1): 38.

Franettovich, M, Chapman, A, Blanch, P, Vicenzino, B (2007b) Augmented low dye tape induced reduction in muscle activation persists following removal of tape. Journal of Science and Medicine in Sport 10(suppl 1): 45.

Franettovich, M, Chapman, A, Vicenzino, B (2008) Tape that increases medial longitudinal arch height also reduces leg muscle activity: a preliminary study. Medicine, Science in Sports, Exercise, 40(4): 593–600.

Fu, T C, Wong, A M, Pei, Y C, Wu, K P, Chou, S W, Lin, Y C (2008) Effect of Kinesio taping on muscle strength in athletes-a pilot study. Journal of Science, Medicine in Sport, 11(2): 198–201.

Fumich, R M, Ellison, A E, Guerin, G J, Grace, P D (1981) The measured effect of taping on combined foot and ankle motion before and after exercise. The American Journal of Sports Medicine, 9(3): 165–70.

Galland, W (1940) An adhesive strapping for sprain of the ankle. Journal of Bone and Joint Surgery American Volume, 22(1): 211–15.

Gibney, V (1895) Sprained ankle: a treatment that involves no loss of time, requires no crutches, and is not attended with an ultimate impairment of function. New York Medical Journal, 61: 193–7.

Gigante, A, Pasquinelli, F M, Paladini, P, Ulisse, S, Greco, F (2001) The effects of patellar taping on patellofemoral incongruence. The American Journal of Sports Medicine, 29(1): 88–92.

Gilleard, W, McConnell, J, Parsons, D (1998) The effect of patellar taping on the onset of vastus medialis obliquus and vastus lateralis muscle activity in persons with patellofemoral pain. Physical Therapy, 78(1): 25–32.

Gray, S D (1991) Sports strapping and bandaging. Australian Family Physician, 20(3): 273, 276–82.

Greene, T A, Hillman, S K (1990) Comparison of support provided by a semirigid orthosis and adhesive ankle taping before, during, and after exercise. The American Journal of Sports Medicine, 18(5): 498–506.

Greig, A M, Bennell, K L, Briggs, A M, Hodges, P W (2008) Postural taping decreases thoracic kyphosis but does not influence trunk muscle electromyographic activity or balance in women with osteoporosis. Manual Therapy, 13, 249–57.

Griffin, A, Bernhardt, J (2006) Strapping the hemiplegic shoulder prevents development of pain during rehabilitation: a randomized controlled trial. Clinical Rehabilitation, 287–95.

Gross, M, Batten, A, Lamm, A, Lorren, J, Stevens, J, Davis, M, Wilkerson, G B (1994) Comparison of DonJoy Ankle Ligament Protector and subtalar sling ankle taping in restricting foot and ankle motion before and after exercise. Journal of Orthopaedic, Sports Physical Therapy, 19(1): 33–41.

Gross, M, Lapp, K, Davis, M (1991) Comparison of Swede-O-Universal® ankle support and Aircast® Sport-Stirrup™ orthoses and ankle tape in restricting eversion-inversion before and after exercise. Journal of Orthopaedic, Sports Physical Therapy, 13(1).

Harradine, P, Herrington, L, Wright, R (2001) The effect of low dye taping upon rear foot motion and position before and after exercise. The Foot, 11(2): 57–60.

Heit, E, Lephart, S, Rozzi, S (1996) The effect of ankle bracing and taping on joint position sense in the stable ankle. Journal of Sport Rehab 5(3): 2013–216.

Herrington, L, Payton, C (1997) Effects of corrective taping of the patella on patients with patellofemoral pain. Physiotherapy, 83(11): 566–72.

Hetherington, B (1996) Lateral ligament strains of the ankle: do they exist? Manual Therapy, 1(5): 274–5.

Hinman, R S, Crossley, K M, McConnell, J, Bennell, K L (2004) Does the application of tape influence quadriceps sensorimotor function in knee osteoarthritis? Rheumatology, 43(3): 331–6.

Horton, S (2002) Acute locked thoracic spine: treatment with a modified SNAG. Manual Therapy, 7(2): 103–7.

Host, H H (1995) Scapular taping in the treatment of anterior shoulder impingement. Physical Therapy, 75(9): 803–12.

Hunt, E, Short, S (2006) Collegiate athletes' perceptions of adhesive ankle taping: a qualitative analysis ' Journal of Sports Rehabilitation, 15(4): 280–98.

Hyland, M, Webber-Gaffney, A, Cohen, L, Lichtman, S (2006) Randomized controlled trial of calcaneal taping, sham taping, and plantar fascia stretching for the short-term management of plantar heel pain. Journal of Orthopaedic, Sports Physical Therapy, 36(6): 364–71.

Jamali, B, Walker, M, Hoke, B, Echternach, J (2004) Windlass taping technique for symptomatic relief of plantar fasciitis. Journal of Sports Rehabilitation, 13(3): 228–43.

Karlsson, J, Andreasson, G O (1992) The effect of external ankle support in chronic lateral ankle joint instability. The American Journal of Sports Medicine, 20(3): 257–61.

Karwoski, A, Plaut, R (2004) Experiments on peeling adhesive tapes from human forearms. Skin Research and Technology, 10(4): 271–7.

Keet, J H L, Gray, J, Harley, Y, Lambert, M I (2007) The effect of medial patellar taping on pain, strength and neuromuscular recruitment in subjects with and without patellofemoral pain. Physiotherapy, 45–52.

Kneeshaw, D (2002) Shoulder taping in the clinical setting. Journal of Bodywork and Movement Therapies, 6(1): 2–8.

Koval, K, Egol, K, Polatsch, D, Baskies, M, Homman, J, Hiebert, R (2003) Tape blisters following hip surgery A prospective, randomized study of two types of tape. Journal of Bone and Joint Surgery American Volume, 85-A(10): 1884–7.

Kowall, M G, Kolk, G, Nuber, G W, Cassisi, J E, Stern, S H (1996) Patellar Taping in the Treatment of Patellofemoral Pain. The American Journal of Sports Medicine, 24(1): 61–6.

Larsen, B, Andreasen, E, Urfer, A, Mickelson, M R, Newhouse, K E (1995) Patellar taping: a radiographic examination of the medial glide technique. The American Journal of Sports Medicine, 23(4): 465–71.

Laughman, R K, Carr, T A, Chao, E Y, Youdas, J W, Sim, F H (1980) Three-dimensional kinematics of the taped ankle before and after exercise. The American Journal of Sports Medicine, 8(6): 425–31.

Lewis, J S, Wright, C, Green, A (2005) Subacromial impingement syndrome: the effect of changing posture on shoulder range of movement. The Journal of Orthopaedic and Sports Physical Therapy, 72–87.

Lohrer, H, Alt, W, Gollhofer, A (1999) Neuromuscular properties and functional aspects of taped ankles. The American Journal of Sports Medicine, 27(1): 69–75.

MacGregor, K, Gerlach, S, Mellor, R, Hodges, P W (2005) Cutaneous stimulation from patella tape causes a differential increase in vasti muscle activity in people with patellofemoral pain. Journal of Orthopaedic Research, 23(2): 351–8.

MacKean, L C, Bell, G, Burnham, R S (1995) Prophylactic ankle bracing vs taping — effects on functional performance in female basketball Players. Journal of Orthopaedic, Sports Physical Therapy, 22(2): 77–81.

McCarthy Persson, J U, Fleming, H, Caulfield, B (2009) The effect of a vastus lateralis tape on muscle activity during stair climbing. Manual Therapy, 14(3): 330–7.

McCarthy Persson, J U, Hooper, A C, Fleming, H E (2007) Repeatability of skin displacement and pressure during 'inhibitory' vastus lateralis muscle taping. Manual Therapy, 12(1): 17–21.

McConnell, J (1986) The management of chondromalacia patellae: a long term solution. Australian Journal of Physiotherapy, 32: 215–23.

—— (2000) A novel approach to pain relief pre-therapeutic exercise. Journal of Science, Medicine in Sport, 3(3): 325–34.

—— (2002) Recalcitrant chronic low back and leg pain - a new theory and different approach to management. Manual Therapy, 7(4): 183–92.

McLean, D A (1989) Use of adhesive strapping in sport. British Journal of Sports Medicine 23(3): 147–9.

Meyer, J, Kulig, K, Landal, R (2002) Differential diagnosis and treatment of subcalcaneal heel pain: a case report. Journal of Orthopaedic, Sports Physical Therapy, 32(3): 114–22.

Mickel, T J, Bottoni, C R, Tsuji, G, Chang, K, Baum, L, Tokushige, K A (2006) Prophylactic bracing versus taping for the prevention of ankle sprains in high school athletes: a prospective, randomized trial (Brief record). Journal of Foot and Ankle Surgery, 360–5.

Moiler, K, Hall, T, Robinson, K (2006) The role of fibular tape in the prevention of ankle injury in basketball: a pilot study. Journal of Orthopaedic, Sports Physical Therapy, 36(9): 661–8.

Morin, G, Tiberio, D, Austin, G (1997) The effect of upper trapezius taping on electromyographic activity in the upper and middle trapezius region. Journal of Sports Rehabilitation, 6(4): 309–18.

Morrissey, D (2000) Proprioceptive shoulder taping. Journal of Bodywork and Movement Therapies, 4: 189–94.

Mulligan, B (1999) Manual Therapy 'NAGS', 'SNAGS', 'MWMS' etc. Plane View Services Ltd, Wellington.

Myburgh, K, Vaughan, C, Isaacs, S (1984) The effects of ankle guards and taping on joint motion before, during, and after a squash match. The American Journal of Sports Medicine, 12(6): 441–6.

Ng, G Y, Chan, H L (2004) The immediate effects of tension of counterforce forearm brace on neuromuscular performance of wrist extensor muscles in subjects with lateral humeral epicondylosis. The Journal of Orthopaedic and Sports Physical Therapy, 72–8.

O'Brien, T, Vicenzino, B (1998) A study of the effects of Mulligan's mobilization with movement treatment of lateral ankle pain using a case study design. Manual Therapy, 3(2): 78–84.

O'Leary, S, Carroll, M, Mellor, R, Scott, A, Vicenzino, B (2002) The effect of soft tissue deloading tape on thoracic spine pressure pain thresholds in asymptomatic subjects. Manual Therapy, 7(3): 150–3.

Olmstead, L C, Vela, L I, Denegar, C R, Hertel, J (2004) Prophylactic ankle taping and bracing: a numbers-needed-to-treat and cost-benefit analysis. Journal of Athletic Training, 39(1): 95–100.

O'Sullivan, K, Kennedy, N, O'Neill, E, Ni Mhainin, U (2008) The effect of low dye taping on rear foot motion and plantar pressure during the stance phase of gait. BMC Musculoskeletal Disorders 9, Article number 11.

Osborne, H R, Allison, G T, Hanna, C (2006) Treatment of plantar fasciitis by low dye taping and iontophoresis: short term results of a double blinded, randomised, placebo controlled clinical trial of dexamethasone and acetic acid * Commentary. British Journal of Sports Medicine, 40(6): 545–9.

Overington, M, Goddard, D, Hing, W (2006) A critical appraisal and literature critique on the effect of patellar taping: is patellar taping effective in the treatment of patellofemoral pain syndrome? (Provisional abstract). New Zealand Journal of Physiotherapy, 66–80.

Parkhurst, T, Burnett, C (1994) Injury and proprioception in the lower back. Journal of Orthopaedic, Sports Physical Therapy, 19(5): 282–95.

Pfeiffer, R R, Debeliso, M, Shea, K G, Kelley, L, Irmischer, B, Harris, C (2004) Kinematic MRI assessment of McConnell taping before and after exercise. American Journal of Sports Medicine 32(3): 621–8.

Powers, C M, Landel, R, Sosnick, T, Kirby, J, Mengel, K, Cheney, A, Perry, J (1997) The effects of patella taping on stride characteristics and joint motion in subjects with patellofemoral pain. Journal of Orthopaedic, Sports Physical Therapy, 26(6): 286–91.

Radford, J, Burns, J, Buchbinder, R, Landorf, K, Cook, C (2006) The effect of low dye taping on kinematic, kinetic, and electromyographic variables: a systematic review. Journal of Orthopaedic, Sports Physical Therapy, 36(4): 232–41.

Refshauge, K M, Raymond, J, Kilbreath, S L, Pengel, L, Heijnen, I (2009) The effect of ankle taping on detection of inversion-eversion movements in participants with recurrent ankle sprain. The American Journal of Sports Medicine, 37(2): 371–5.

Robbins, S, Waked, E, Rappel, R (1995) Ankle taping improves proprioception before and after exercise in young men. British Journal of Sports Medicine, 29(4): 242–7.

Ryan, C G, Rowe, P J (2006) An electromyographical study to investigate the effects of patellar taping on the vastus medialis/vastus lateralis ratio in asymptomatic participants. Physiotherapy Theory and Practice, 309–15.

Salsich, G B, Brechter, J H et al (2002) The effects of patellar taping on knee kinetics, kinematics, and vastus lateralis muscle activity during stair ambulation in individuals with patellofemoral pain. Journal of Orthopaedic, Sports Physical Therapy, 32(1): 3–10.

Sekar, S, Srinivas, C (2008) Comparative efficacy of soap water, spirit, acetone and ether in removing the adherent material formed during and after removal of Micropore tape. Indian Journal of Dermatology Venereology and Leprology, 74(4): 391–2.

Selkowitz, D M, Chaney, C, Stuckey, S J, Vlad, G (2007) The effects of scapular taping on the surface electromyographic signal amplitude of shoulder girdle muscles during upper extremity elevation in individuals with suspected shoulder impingement syndrome. Journal of Orthopaedic, Sports Physical Therapy, 37(11): 694–702.

Shamus, J L, Shamus, E C (1997) A taping technique for the treatment of acromioclavicular joint sprains: a case study. Journal of Orthopaedic, Sports Physical Therapy, 25(6): 390–4.

Shapiro, M S, Kabo, J M, Mitchell, P W, Loren, G, Tsenter, M (1994) Ankle sprain prophylaxis: an analysis of the stabilizing effects of braces and tape. The American Journal of Sports Medicine 22(1): 78–82.

Shim, Y, Lee, H, Lee, D (2003) The use of elastic adhesive tape to promote lymphatic flow in the rabbit hind leg. Yonsei Medical Journal, 44(6).

Simoneau, G, Degner, R, Kramper, C, Kittleson, K (1997) Changes in ankle joint proprioception resulting from strips of athletic tape applied over the skin. Journal of Athletic Training, 32(2): 141–7.

Slupik, A, Dwornik, M, Bialoszewski, D, Zych, E (2007) Effect of Kinesio Taping on bioelectrical activity of vastus medialis muscle: preliminary report. Ortopedia Traumatologia Rehabilitacja, 9(6): 644–51.

Somes, S, Worrell, T, Corey, B, Ingersoll, C (1997) Effects of patellar taping on patellar position in the open and closed kinetic chain: a preliminary study. Journal of Sports Rehabilitation, 6(4): 299–308.

Stoddard, J K, Johnson, C D (2000) Conservative treatment of a patient with a mild acromioclavicular joint separation. Journal of Sports Chiropractic, Rehabilitation, 14(4): 118–28.

Thacker, S B, Stroup, D F, Branche, C M, Gilchrist, J, Goodman, R A, Weitman, E A (1999) The prevention of ankle sprains in sports. The American Journal of Sports Medicine, 27(6): 753–60.

Thelen, M, Dauber, J, Stoneman, P (2008) The clinical efficacy of Kinesio tape for shoulder pain: a randomised, double-blinded, clinical trial. Journal of Orthopaedic, Sports Physical Therapy, 38(7).

Tokumura, F, Homma, T, Tomiya, T, Kobayashi, Y, Matsuda, T (2007) Properties of pressure-sensitive adhesive tapes with soft adhesives to human skin and their mechanism. Skin Research and Technology, 13(2): 211–16.

Tokumura, F, Umekage, K, Sado, M, Otsuka, S, Suda, S, Taniguchi, M, Yamori, A, Nakamura, A, Kawai, J, Oka, K (2005) Skin irritation due to repetitive application of adhesive tape: the influence of adhesive strength and seasonal variability. Skin Research and Technology, 11(2): 102–6.

Tokumura, F, Yoshiura, Y, Homma, T, Nukatsuka, H (2006) Regional differences in adhesive tape stripping of human skin. Skin Research and Technology, 12(3): 178–82.

Vaes, P, De Boeck, F, Handelberg, F, Opdecam, P (1985) Comparative radiological study of the influence of ankle joint strapping and taping on ankle stability. Journal of Orthopaedic, Sports Physical Therapy, 7(3).

Vicenzino, B (2003) Lateral epicondylalgia: a musculoskeletal physiotherapy perspective. Manual Therapy, 8(2): 66–79.

Vicenzino, B, Brooksbank, J, Minto, J, Offord, S, Paungmali, A (2003) Initial effects of elbow taping on pain-free grip strength and pressure pain threshold. Journal of Orthopaedic, Sports Physical Therapy, 33(7): 400–7.

Vicenzino, B, Franettovich, M, Mcpoil, T, Russell, T, Skardoon, G, Bartold, S J (2005) Initial effects of anti-pronation tape on the medial longitudinal arch during walking and running — commentary. British Journal of Sports Medicine, 39(12): 939–43.

Vicenzino, B, Griffiths, S, Griffiths, L, Hadley, A (2000) Effect of antipronation tape and temporary orthotic on vertical navicular height before and after exercise. Journal of Orthopaedic, Sports Physical Therapy, 30(6).

Vicenzino, B, Mcpoil, T, Buckland, S (2007a) Plantar foot pressures after the augmented low dye taping technique. Journal of Athletic Training, 42(3): 374–80.

Vicenzino, B, Paungmali, A, Teys, P (2007b) Mulligan's mobilization-with-movement, positional faults and pain relief: current concepts from a critical review of literature. Manual Therapy, 12(2): 98–108.

Vicenzino, B, Wright, A (1995) Effects of a novel manipulative physiotherapy technique on tennis elbow: a single case study. Manual Therapy, 1(1): 30–5.

Wildman, T, Oostman, H, Storrs, F (2008) Allergic contact dermatitis from medical adhesive bandages in patients who report having a reaction to medical bandages. Dermatitis 19(1): 32–7.

Wilson, T, Carter, N, Thomas, G (2003) A multicenter, single-masked, study of medial, neutral, and lateral patellar taping in individuals with patellofemoral pain syndrome. Journal of Orthopaedic, Sports Physical Therapy, 33(8): 437–43.

Worrell, T, Ingersoll, C D, Bockrath-Pugliese, K, Minis, P (1998) Effect of patellar taping and bracing on patellar position as determined by MRI in patients with patellofemoral pain. Journal of Athletic Training, 33(1): 16–20.

CHAPTER 3

Precautions and preparation procedures

The main aims of this chapter are to review specific precautions and contraindications to taping, to discuss patient preparation for taping and to outline the main materials required for taping. Commonly used tips for the effective application of tape are also included in this chapter.

PRECAUTIONS IN TAPING

Adhesive tape may cause adverse effects in some people. Generally tape should not be used in cases where the patient has:
○ skin allergy or sensitivity to tape
○ open wounds
○ skin infections and/or conditions (e.g. dermatitis, eczema)
○ fragile or sensitive skin in the area to be taped, which is prone to tears and bruising
○ circulatory conditions — bleeding or clotting disorders
○ sensory loss around the area to be taped, or distal to the taped area.

Precaution should be exercised when using tape on people with:
○ peripheral vascular disease
○ peripheral neuropathies
○ diabetes
○ prolonged use of steroid or anticoagulant medication
○ cognitive loss where the patient is unable to report possible side-effects of taping.

Regardless of whether or not a patient has a known sensitivity to tape the therapist needs to be aware that patients may develop skin irritation with prolonged or repeated use of tape application and removal (Tokumura et al 2005). Also, in some people adhesive tapes can cause adhesive contact (ACD) dermatitis or irritant contact dermatitis (ICD) (Wildman, Oostman & Storrs 2008). Another consideration is that the skin may be more sensitive immediately after shaving and if possible taping should be avoided immediately after shaving.

If a patient develops ACD or ICD during or after tape application, the tape and any adhesive residue should be removed completely, and following removal cold water can be used to cool the area. If the irritation does not settle, is painful, or the skin has broken down, the patient should be referred for medical assessment and management.

An example of a skin reaction due to adhesive tape is shown in Figure 2.2 on page 23.

PATIENT WARNINGS AND CONSENT

Pre-taping informed consent and precautions

Consistent with standard clinical practice and for the intention of gaining informed consent prior to the application of any taping techniques, the therapist must explain to the patient the purpose of the technique, what it involves, the expected outcomes, potential risks, alternative treatments to taping and allow the patient to ask any questions. Prior to applying tape, to help exclude the possibility that the patient has any known allergy to adhesive materials, the therapist should ask the patient:

Do you have any known allergy or sensitivity to tape, bandaids or other adhesive material?

If the patient is not aware of any known allergy or sensitivity to tape the therapist may still prefer to apply a small 25 mm strip of rigid tape near the area to be taped for 20 minutes for the purpose of determining if the patient demonstrates a skin reaction, redness, itchiness or irritability to tape.

Post-taping precautions and warnings

During and after each application of a taping technique the therapist must ensure that:

1 the taping technique is comfortable with no feelings of restriction, tightness or pain
2 the patient is questioned to check if they are experiencing pins and needles, numbness or other symptoms of impaired circulation
3 circulation is present by inspecting the site of the tape for signs of occlusion, such as:
   a skin changes of pallor, redness or cyanosis
   b oedema or swelling around the tape area

c reduced capillary return, as tested by applying a gentle pressure to the skin distal to the tape and watching for the capillary return on removal of the gentle pressure
d reduced pulse
4 the tape application is inspected closely and has no creases or folds to cause discomfort
5 the tape application is checked passively where necessary to confirm available passive range of motion (ROM)
6 the aims and objectives for which the tape was applied are met through using relevant outcome measures, as discussed in Chapter 1 and in each technique.

The therapist should give an appropriate standard warning regarding the precautions of taping at the completion of each taping technique, before the patient's departure. A detailed example of a warning may include:

You may leave the tape on for up to 48 hours. The tape can become wet if you wish to swim or shower with it on. However, you must ensure the tape is adequately dry prior to being covered. If at any time you are experiencing:
• additional discomfort
• increase in any of your symptoms
• feelings of pins and needles or numbness at the site of the tape, around the area of the tape or below the area being taped
• feelings of skin itchiness or irritability under the tape
• skin colour changes around the tape such as pallor, redness or blueness
• skin temperature changes, such as a feeling of coldness or hot to touch or increased swelling around the tape
then you must remove the tape immediately. The tape can be removed by folding it back on itself as shown to you, and using a

pair of scissors to cut the tape off after lifting it away from your body. The tape can also be removed using eucalyptus oil if you have no allergy to this. If you have any concerns regarding the application and removal of this taping technique please feel free to contact me. Do you understand this warning? Do you have any questions?'

The therapist may wish to incorporate in their practice the use of a standard consent and information sheet on taping which includes the above warning. A copy of the information sheet may be given to the patient. A sample information sheet with warnings and consent information is included in Appendix 2.

TAPING MATERIALS

The main materials (Fig 3.1) needed to perform all taping techniques in this book are:

○ required materials:
   • rigid adhesive tape, usually 38 mm width
   • hypoallergenic underlay adhesive tape, 5 cm width
   • blunt nose scissors
   • shavers or hair clippers for hair removal
   • strong fingers with short nails
○ optional materials:
   • thin foam under-wrap to be used under rigid sports tape
   • elasticised bandage tape to over-wrap rigid sports tape
   • elasticised narrow tape for finger and toe taping
   • skin preparation spray
   • adhesive spray
   • Friars' Balsam to increase tape adhesion
   • eucalyptus oil or commercial tape solvent for removing tape.

There are several rigid adhesive tapes available in the market and they may exhibit varying characteristics such as tensile strength,

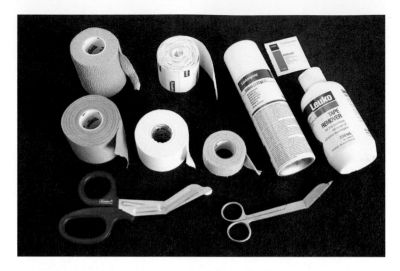

FIGURE 3.1 TAPING MATERIALS — HYPOALLERGENIC UNDERLAY TAPE, FOAM UNDER-WRAP, ADHESIVE SPRAY, BLUNT NOSE SCISSORS

conformity and adhesiveness (Bragg et al 2002; Beringer 2008). Cost and availability of tape may vary in different countries and care must be taken when selecting tape to ensure it has adequate adhesiveness and conformity without jeopardising the tensile strength to ensure the techniques are performed effectively. The tape is torn usually using fingers. The therapist tenses the tape at the desired length, and with one hand stabilises the tape edge with the thumb and flexed index finger and using the thumb and flexed index finger of the other hand tears the tape quickly in a horizontal and opposite direction (Fig 3.2). In a similar fashion the tape can be torn longitudinally when thin strips of tape are needed for certain techniques. Alternatively the tape can be cut using blunt nose scissors.

There are various brands of hypoallergenic underlay, but

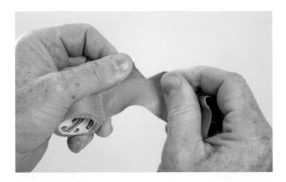

FIGURE 3.2 FINGER POSITION FOR RIPPING TAPE

generally it is manufactured from a stretchable non-woven tape with a breathable porous adhesive material. It is commonly produced with a paper backing. The therapist needs to familiarise themselves with removing the paper backing prior to application to ensure speedy efficient application. The hypoallergenic underlay is not designed to be able to be torn by hand and needs to be cut using scissors.

PREPARATION FOR TAPE APPLICATION

To enable efficiency and precision in the application of any taping technique the treatment area and the patient need to be adequately prepared using the following steps.

1 The tape should be applied on dry clean skin to reduce the risk of skin irritation and to improve tape adhesiveness.
2 Any underlying body hair may be removed using either a shaver or electric hair clippers.
3 Hypoallergenic underlay adhesive tape may be applied under the rigid tape in areas where the rigid tape causes increased traction on the skin, or where the patient has a known sensitivity to tape.

4 For sensitive skin the use of under-wrap foam may be applied under the tape to reduce the adhesive reaction from the tape. However, non-adhesive under-wrapping can reduce the effectiveness of some taping techniques due to slippage.
5 In some countries adhesive spray or skin preparation sprays may be available, and these may be sprayed on the skin prior to taping to increase tape adhesion. Friars' Balsam (tincture of benzoin) is also a product easily obtained from a pharmacy that may be applied under tape to increase tape adhesion (Beringer 2008).

APPLICATION OF TAPE

For all techniques the therapist should first ensure:
○ the patient is in a comfortable and safe position in preparation for the tape application
○ the limb, joint or body area to be taped is adequately exposed and is placed in the ideal required position for the effective application of the specific technique
○ the therapist's position is ergonomically efficient and safe.

As discussed in Chapter 1, excellent knowledge of anatomy of the area to be taped is required by the therapist to ensure success of the taping technique and safety of the patient.

Some general tips useful in the application of tape are provided below.
○ Use proximal and distal anchors (Fig 3.3) as required, to enable following tape strips to be attached as necessary.
○ Apply tape from distal to proximal direction where possible.
○ Tension the tape and while maintaining the tension apply the tape with even pressure, laying it down on the skin, rather than pulling it into the skin, to avoid compromising circulation.
○ When applying tape around limbs, particularly anchors and

closing lock-offs, ask the patient to contract their muscles during tape application.

○ Apply tape around body contours and bony areas by allowing the tape to follow the natural direction of the body contour. Do not force tape to change direction.

○ Avoid transverse circumferential tape, particularly for techniques where the tape ends meet. Tape placed around limbs should be placed in slight oblique orientation to avoid compromising the circulation (Fig 3.4).

○ Avoid continuous taping; rather, use one circle of tape at a time.

○ Where required by the technique the tape may overlap the previous strip of tape by half its width (Fig 3.5).

○ When applying tape ensure application is smooth, with no tape creases or folds, as these may cause skin pressure with the potential to become painful.

○ Apply lock-off strips of tape at the completion of the technique to stabilise the strips of tape already in place.

REMOVAL OF TAPE

Tape can be removed by the therapist or by patients themselves after they have been instructed on the process. Some tips on removing tape are provided below.

○ In applications using multiple layers of tape, blunt nose scissors may be used to cut the tape.

○ Where possible tape should be folded back on itself and slowly removed from the skin with one hand while the other hand gently applies pressure on the skin in the opposite direction. Karwoski and Plaut (2004) found that peel force on the skin was at a minimum when the tape was peeled off at an angle of 150°, and when the tape was peeled slowly (Fig 3.6). They concluded that reducing peel force reduces the likelihood of pain and trauma during tape removal (Karwoski & Plaut 2004).

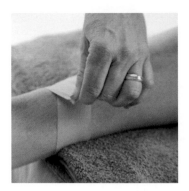

FIGURE 3.3 ANCHOR TAPE

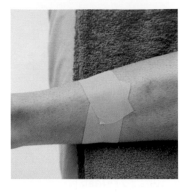

FIGURE 3.4 OBLIQUE ORIENTATION OF CIRCUMFERENTIAL TAPE (IN AN ANCHOR)

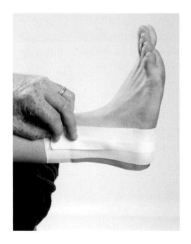

FIGURE 3.5 OVERLAPPING TAPE BY HALF THE PREVIOUS WIDTH

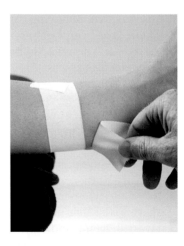

FIGURE 3.6 PEELING TAPE OFF BY FOLDING IT BACK ON ITSELF AT 150°

- Eucalyptus oil can be used as a solvent for the removal of tape adhesive.
- Commercially produced adhesive solvents may be available on the market, but care needs to be taken when using these.

REFERENCES

Beringer, R (2008) Study of the adhesiveness of medical tapes when wet, dry or following application of Friars' Balsam. Paediatric Anaesthesia, 18(6): 520–4.

Bragg, R W, MacMahon, J M, Overom, E K, Yerby, S A, Matheson, G O, Carter, D R, Andriacchi, T P (2002) Failure and fatigue characteristics of adhesive athletic tape. Medicine and Science in Sports and Exercise, 34(3): 403–10.

Karwoski, A, Plaut, R (2004) Experiments on peeling adhesive tapes from human forearms. Skin Research and Technology, 10(4): 271–7.

Tokumura, F, Umekage, K, Sado, M, Otsuka, S, Suda, S, Taniguchi, M, Yamori, A, Nakamura, A, Kawai, J, Oka, K (2005) Skin irritation due to repetitive application of adhesive tape: the influence of adhesive strength and seasonal variability. Skin Research and Technology, 11(2): 102–6.

Wildman, T, Oostman, H, Storrs, F (2008) Allergic contact dermatitis from medical adhesive bandages in patients who report having a reaction to medical bandages. Dermatitis, 19(1): 32–7.

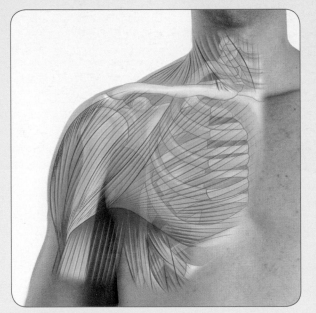

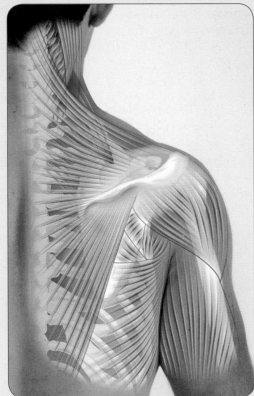

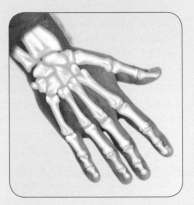

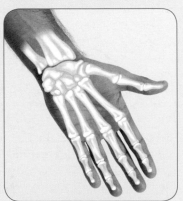

Scapula

Scapula position — postural

Overview, background and rationale

Sustained forward posture position with altered scapula mechanics may be a contributing or concomitant factor to shoulder, neck, thoracic spine and other related upper limb conditions (Peterson et al 1997; Pascarelli & Hsu 2001). Altered scapula muscle activity such as increased motor activity of pectoralis minor and levator scapulae muscles, and decreased motor activity of serratus anterior and lower trapezius muscles may further encourage scapula malposition (Sahrmann 2002; Lewis & Valentine 2007) as would thoracic spine kyphosis.

Scapula position and scapular muscle activation is often incorporated in the assessment and management of shoulder, neck, thoracic spine and other upper limb conditions (Donatelli 2004). Taping has been postulated to facilitate muscles with decreased motor activity and/or inhibit overactive muscles or to maintain the ideal scapula position as part of the therapeutic approach to managing these predisposing factors to upper limb or spinal conditions (Lewis et al 2005; Selkowitz et al 2007; Greig et al 2008).

The scapula and postural taping techniques studied in the literature do not all use a standard technique and do not all use the same type of tape. Similarly, taping techniques used by therapists vary considerably. This makes comparison of the findings in the literature difficult. A discussion of the studies on the relevant scapular taping techniques investigated in the literature or techniques commonly used by therapists is included in Chapter 2.

The following techniques are aimed at facilitating awareness of corrected scapula position and improving postural control. Where indicated, techniques are varied slightly to address and alter concomitant problems such as anterior head of humerus (HOH) position, overactive pectoralis minor or overactive levator scapulae and/or upper trapezius muscles. Techniques on the scapulae are usually applied bilaterally. However, if only one side of the scapulohumeral region is symptomatic and requires a specific therapeutic application as described in techniques 1–4 this may be utilised on the symptomatic side, while a standard postural taping technique as described in technique 1 may be applied to the non-symptomatic side.

Postural-position scapula

Background and rationale

This technique addresses the scapula position although it has also been shown to assist in decreasing thoracic kyphosis (Greig et al 2008). It is aimed at applying tape over the scapula in the desired preset position to increase patient awareness when correcting their posture and to facilitate appropriate scapular muscular activation.

Evidence

- Postural tape may be effective in reducing kyphosis (Greig et al 2008) (Level IV).
- Scapulae tape decreases upper trapezius muscle activity in subjects with shoulder pain (Selkowitz et al 2007) (Level IV).

Material

- Hypoallergenic underlay 2 × 40–50 cm strips.
- Rigid tape 2 × 40–50 cm strips.

Patient position

- Patient sits with feet well supported and pelvis in neutral position. Arms are either placed with shoulder in neutral position or resting on a pillow in 30° shoulder abduction.
- Patient aims to actively set their scapulae in the position prescribed by the therapist.

Therapist position

- Therapist stands beside or behind the patient.
- Therapist further assists the scapulae in the prescribed position.

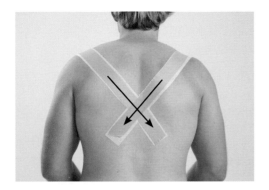
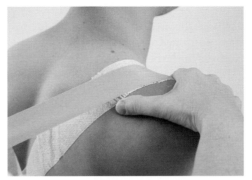

1 Apply hypoallergenic underlay starting anterior to the glenohumeral (GH) joint line.
2 Direct hypoallergenic underlay posteriorly and diagonally over the scapula, crossing the spine at about the T6 spinous process and finishing on the contralateral side approximately in line with T8–T10 spinous processes.
3 Steps 1 and 2 are repeated with hypoallergenic underlay for the contralateral side.
4 Apply tape over hypoallergenic underlay starting anterior to the GH joint line. Tension the tape and while maintaining the tension lay it down gently over the hypoallergenic underlay.
5 Step 5 is repeated on the contralateral side.

Reassessment
○ Posture.
○ Position of scapula(e).
○ Upper limb, cervical or thoracic spine provocative movement and symptom presentation.
○ Provocative functional task.

Scapula position with correction of head of humerus (HOH) position

Background and rationale

In anterior shoulder impingement, symptoms may be associated with forward protracted scapula with an anteriorly positioned HOH (Donatelli 2004). Taping may be used to address both the scapula and the HOH position simultaneously. This technique addresses the scapula position as above (technique 1) while at the same time incorporating an antero-posterior glide on an anteriorly placed HOH (discussed in the next section in technique 10).

Evidence

O Tape may be used to address scapula position (Selkowitz et al 2007; Greig et al 2008) (Level IV).
O Tape may be used to address humeral head position but published works are clinical or anecdotal reports (Hess 2000; McConnell 2000) (Clinical reports).

Material

O Hypoallergenic underlay 2 × 40–50 cm strips.
O Rigid tape 2 × 40–50 cm strips.

Patient position

O Patient sits with feet well supported and pelvis in neutral position. Arms are either placed with shoulder in neutral position or resting on a pillow in 30° shoulder abduction.
O Patient aims to actively set their scapulae in the position prescribed by the therapist.

Therapist position

O Therapist stands beside or behind the patient.
O Therapist further assists the scapulae in the prescribed position.

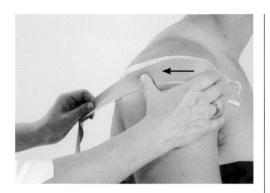 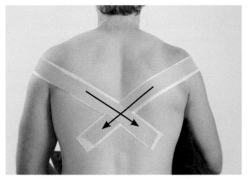 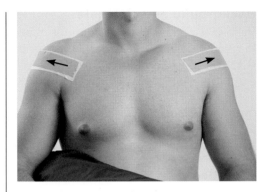

1 Apply hypoallergenic underlay starting anterior to the GH joint.
2 Direct hypoallergenic underlay over the lateral aspect of the upper humerus and diagonally over the scapula, aiming to lay the hypoallergenic underlay gently along the lower trapezius muscle fibres.
3 Step 1 can be repeated for the non-affected side.
4 Apply the tape over the hypo-allergenic underlay, anterior to the GH joint, and bring the tape over the lateral aspect of the upper humerus.
5 Tension the tape with one hand and perform an antero-posterior glide to the HOH with the other hand while laying the tensioned tape over the hypoallergenic underlay.

6 Lay the tape over the direction of the lower trapezius muscle fibres gently. This may assist in increased patient awareness of the lower trapezius muscle activation in scapula control.

7 Apply tape over the hypoallergenic underlay on the non-affected scapula, starting anterior to the GH joint, repeating steps 4 and 5, without applying the antero-posterior glide on the HOH unless so indicated in the assessment.

Reassessment

○ Posture.
○ Position of scapula(e).
○ Upper limb, cervical or thoracic spine provocative movement and symptom presentation.
○ Provocative functional task.

Scapula position for postural correction, with pectoralis minor 'stretch'

Background and rationale

Increased motor activity or tightness of pectoralis minor muscle may present in patients with shoulder or postural problems (Lewis & Valentine 2007). This taping technique combines the scapula position taping (technique 1) in a modified application to apply a 'stretch' on the pectoralis minor muscle. The tape starts over the coracoid process, the anatomic insertion of the pectoralis minor muscle, prior to applying it on the scapula. It may be a useful technique to correct posture involving protracted scapulae.

Evidence

○ Tape may be applied to address scapula position and posture (Greig et al 2008).
○ No research studies relating to this technique were identified.

Material

○ Hypoallergenic underlay 2 × 40–50 cm strips.
○ Rigid tape 2 × 40–50 cm strips.

Patient position

○ Patient sits with feet well supported and pelvis in neutral position. Arms are either placed with shoulder in neutral position or resting on a pillow in 30° shoulder abduction.
○ Patient aims to actively set their scapulae in the position prescribed by the therapist.

Therapist position

○ Therapist stands beside or behind the patient.
○ Therapist further assists the scapulae in the prescribed position.

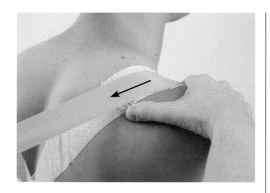

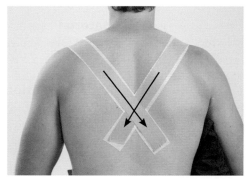

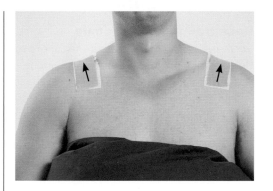

1 Apply hypoallergenic underlay starting anterior to the GH joint, approximately 2 cm below the coracoid process.

2 Bring the hypoallergenic underlay superiorly to the shoulder, across the spine of the scapula, aiming to lay hypoallergenic underlay along the lower trapezius muscle fibres.

3 Steps 1 and 2 can be repeated for the non-affected scapula side.

4 Start the tape over the hypoallergenic underlay, anterior to the GH joint, approximately 2 cm below the coracoid process.

5 With one hand perform gentle posterior tilt glide on the scapula while applying the tensioned tape with the other hand.

6 Lay the tape over the direction of the lower trapezius muscle fibres gently. This may increase patient awareness of the lower trapezius muscle to assist in its activation.

7 The therapist may apply tape over hypoallergenic underlay on the non-affected scapula, starting anterior and superior to the GH joint as described in steps 4 and 6 without performing the posterior tilt glide on the scapula.

Reassessment

○ Posture position.
○ Position of scapula(e).
○ Upper limb, cervical or thoracic spine provocative movement and symptom presentation
○ Provocative functional task.

Scapula position with upper trapezius/levator scapulae deloading/inhibition

Background and rationale

Scapula dyskinesis as a result of scapula muscle dysfunction may be identified in the assessment of patients with neck, shoulder or thoracic pain (Kibler 2006). Upper trapezius is one of the scapular muscles that has been reported to have increased activity in chronic neck pain (Falla, Bilenkij & Jull 2004) and in shoulder pain conditions (Selkowitz et al 2007). This taping technique addresses the scapula position as in technique 1, while incorporating a deloading effect on the upper trapezius and/or levator scapulae muscles, encouraging decrease in the activity of these muscles with scapula motion.

Evidence

○ Selkowitz et al (2007) found that upper trapezius activity is reduced by scapula taping in subjects with shoulder pain (Level IV).
○ Morin et al (1997) found that tape placed over the upper trapezius decreased upper trapezius activity in uninjured subjects during a scapula stabilisation task (Level IV).

Material

○ Hypoallergenic underlay 2 × 40–50 cm strips.
○ Rigid tape 2 × 40–50 cm strips.

Patient position

○ Patient sits with feet well supported and pelvis in neutral position. Arms are either placed by the side with shoulder in neutral position or resting on a pillow in 30° shoulder abduction.
○ Patient aims to actively set their scapulae in the position prescribed by the therapist.

Therapist position

○ Therapist stands beside or behind the patient.
○ Therapist further assists the scapulae in the prescribed position.

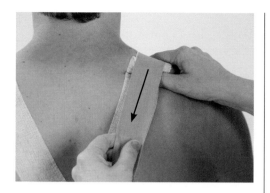
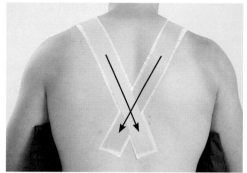
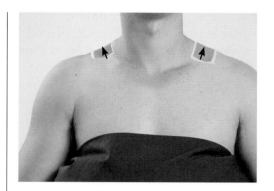

1 Apply hypoallergenic underlay starting anterior and superior to the clavicle and below the mid region of the upper trapezius muscle fibres.

2 Bring hypoallergenic underlay perpendicular to the direction of the upper trapezius (and/or levator scapula) muscle fibres, laying it along the direction of the lower trapezius muscle fibres to finish at approximately the contralateral transverse processes of T9–T11.

3 Step 1 is repeated for the non-affected scapula.

4 Start the tape over the hypoallergenic underlay anterior and superior to the clavicle. Using a lumbrical grip, gather and hold the upper trapezius and/or levator scapulae muscle across its fibre direction with one hand, tension and lay the tape over the hypo-allergenic underlay with the other hand.

5 Step 3 is repeated on the contralateral scapula. If deloading is not required on the contralateral scapula an option is to apply the tape over the hypoallergenic underlay without applying the deloading effect on the upper trapezius levator scapulae muscle.

Reassessment

○ Posture position.
○ Position of scapula(e).
○ Upper limb, cervical or thoracic spine provocative movement and symptom presentation.
○ Provocative functional task.

Upper trapezius/levator scapulae deloading/inhibition

Background and rationale

Upper trapezius is one of the scapular muscles that has been reported to have increased activity in chronic neck pain (Falla et al 2004) and in shoulder pain conditions (Selkowitz et al 2007). In treatment it may be necessary to address this upper trapezius overactivity. This taping technique focuses on the inhibition effect of a deloading technique on the upper trapezius and/or levator scapulae to reduce the overactivity of these muscles.

Evidence

○ Selkowitz et al (2007) found that upper trapezius activity is reduced by scapula taping in subjects with shoulder pain (Level IV).
○ Morin et al (1997) found that tape placed over the upper trapezius muscle decreased its activity in uninjured subjects during a scapula stabilisation task (Level IV).

Material

○ Hypoallergenic underlay 2 × 10–15 cm strips.
○ Rigid tape 2 × 10–15 cm strips.

Patient position

○ Patient sits with feet well supported and pelvis in neutral position. Arms are either placed with shoulder in neutral position or resting on a pillow in 30° shoulder abduction.
○ Patient actively sets their scapulae in the position prescribed by the therapist.

Therapist position

○ Therapist stands beside or behind the patient.
○ Therapist further assists the scapulae in the prescribed position.

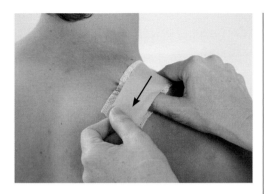

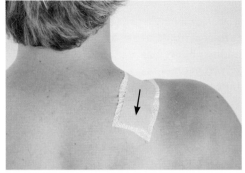

1 Apply hypoallergenic underlay starting anterior and superior to the clavicle and anterior to the upper trapezius muscle fibres. Bring hypoallergenic underlay perpendicular to the orientation of the upper trapezius muscle fibres and finish about 1 cm below the upper trapezius fibres on the posterior aspect. If the aim is to incorporate levator scapulae muscle in this technique, finish the hypoallergenic underlay inferior and medial to the levator scapulae muscle insertion on the superior medial angle of the scapula.

2 Step 1 can be repeated for the contralateral side if applying the technique bilaterally.

3 Start the tape over the hypoallergenic underlay, anterior to the upper trapezius muscle fibres. Gather and hold the upper trapezius and/or levator scapulae muscle across the fibre orientation using a 'lumbrical' grip with one hand and apply the tape with the other hand, laying it over the hypoallergenic underlay.

4 Step 3 can be repeated for the contralateral side if applying the technique bilaterally.

Reassessment
○ Patient comfort and symptom presentation at rest.
○ Resting tone of upper trapezius and/or levator scapulae muscle.
○ Position of scapula and scapula setting exercise.
○ Upper limb, cervical or thoracic spine provocative movement and symptom presentation.

5

Lower trapezius muscle facilitation

Background and rationale

Decreased activity of lower trapezius muscle may be associated with altered scapula mechanics and it is thought to contribute to increased scapula elevation. The following technique follows the proposed effects of tape in facilitating muscle activation described in Chapter 2 (p 25). A single strip of tape is applied over the muscle along the fibre orientation. It aims to apply a tactile facilitation to the muscle, increasing patient awareness and subsequent activation. Anatomy knowledge of the muscle is very important; lower trapezius muscle origin is from spinous processes of T6–T12 and insertion is on the apex of the spine of the scapula.

Evidence

- Selkowitz et al (2007) found that tape applied over the upper trapezius and extending over the lower trapezius did increase lower trapezius electromyography (EMG) activity in patients with shoulder pain (Level IV).
- Alexander et al (2003) found that the tape decreased lower trapezius muscle activity during its application in healthy subjects (Level IV).

Material

- Hypoallergenic underlay 1×15–25 cm strip (optional).
- Rigid tape 1×15–25 cm strip.

Patient position

- Patient sits with feet well supported and pelvis in neutral position. Arms are either placed with shoulder in neutral position or resting on a pillow in 30° shoulder abduction.
- Patient aims to actively set their scapulae in the position prescribed by the therapist.

Therapist position

- Therapist stands beside or behind the patient.
- Therapist further assists the scapulae in the prescribed position.

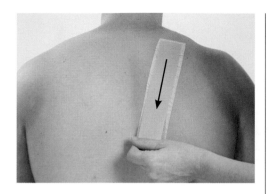

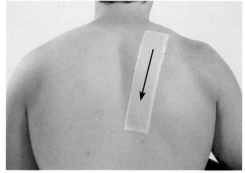

1   Lightly apply hypoallergenic underlay starting at the medial apex of the spine of the scapula. Lay the hypoallergenic underlay in the same direction as the lower trapezius muscle fibres, finishing near the insertion of the lower trapezius muscle at the spinous process of T12.

2   Apply the tape very lightly over the hypoallergenic underlay following the same direction. Ensure no added pressure is exerted while applying the tape.

Reassessment
○ Patient comfort and symptom presentation at rest.
○ Position of scapula.
○ Therapeutic exercise for lower trapezius muscle (scapula setting exercise).
○ Upper limb, cervical or thoracic spine provocative movement and symptom presentation.

6

Serratus anterior muscle facilitation

Background and rationale

Scapula dyskinesis as a result of scapula muscle dysfunction may be concomitant to shoulder pathology (Kibler 2006) with weakness or dysfunction of the serratus anterior muscle being one of the associated assessment findings. The following technique follows the muscle facilitatory principles described in Chapter 2. A single strip of tape is applied over the muscle in line with the muscle fibre orientation. The aim is for the tape to increase patient awareness and subsequent activation of the muscle. Anatomy knowledge of the muscle is very important; serratus anterior origin is from anterior ribs 1–8 and insertion is on the medial border of the scapula.

Evidence

- Morrissey (2000) presented a similar technique in a clinical report proposing it increases activity of the muscle through stimulation of subcutaneous mechanoreceptors (Clinical report).
- No research studies relating to this technique were identified.

Material

- Hypoallergenic underlay 1 × 20–25 cm strip (optional).
- Rigid tape 1 × 20–25 cm strip.

Patient position

- Patient sits with feet well supported and pelvis in neutral position.
- Patient aims to actively set their scapulae in the position prescribed by the therapist.
- The arm may be in 30° shoulder abduction, resting on a pillow, or placed in the flexion position at which range the patient loses their scapula control.

Therapist position

- Therapist stands beside or behind the patient.
- Therapist further assists the scapulae in the prescribed position.

7

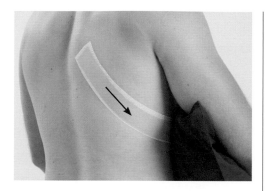

1 Lightly apply hypoallergenic underlay starting at the medial border of the scapula near the insertion of serratus anterior. Bring the tape over the serratus anterior, aligning it in the same direction as the muscle fibres, and finish the tape near the serratus anterior origin on ribs 1–8 anteriorly.

2 Apply the tape very lightly over the hypoallergenic underlay, following the same orientation. Ensure no added pressure is exerted while applying the tape.

Reassessment

○ Position of scapula at rest and with upper limb movement.
○ Serratus anterior control druing therapeutic exercise or functional tasks.

7

Scapula stabilisation in long thoracic nerve palsy

Background and rationale
Long thoracic nerve palsy can cause paralysis or substantial weakness of the serratus anterior muscle, leading to obvious scapula winging (Lorei & Hershman 1993). This can have a detrimental effect on scapula control and stability and subsequently effect the function of the affected upper limb. Bracing has been used previously in long thoracic nerve palsy cases to support the scapula (Marin 1998). In the absence of appropriate bracing taping can be used to provide mechanical support to the scapula and proprioceptive input to the stabilising muscles, in particular the affected serratus anterior. This technique addresses the scapula position and involves applying tape around the scapula in the desired position to provide some support for the affected scapula until muscle activation necessary to maintain the position is returned.

Evidence
- Marin (1998) found that bracing to decrease scapula winging reported decreased shoulder pain and increased shoulder motion (Level IV).
- No research studies relating to this taping technique were identified.

Material
- Hypoallergenic underlay 3 × 20–25 cm strips.
- Rigid tape 3–6 × 2–25 cm strips.

Patient position
- Patient sits with feet well supported and pelvis in neutral position.
- Patient aims to actively set their scapulae in the position prescribed by the therapist.
- The arm may be in 30° shoulder abduction, resting on a pillow, or placed in the flexion position at which range the patient loses their scapula control.

Therapist position
- Therapist stands beside or behind the patient.
- Therapist further assists the scapulae in the prescribed position.

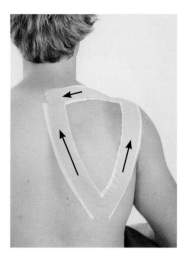

1 Apply hypoallergenic underlay around the scapula; one strip applied along the medial border of the scapula, from the inferior to the superior scapular angle, one strip applied from the inferior angle along the lateral border of the scapula and one strip applied superiorly from the GH joint to the cervico-thoracic junction. The three strips of hypoallergenic underlay join each other.

2 Apply three strips of tensioned tape over hypoallergenic underlay following the landmarks in step 1.

Reassessment

○ Position of scapula at rest and during active upper limb motion — observe if scapula is winging.

○ Serratus anterior activation therapeutic exercise.

○ Upper limb, cervical or thoracic spine provocative movement.

8

Deloading in thoracic outlet syndrome

Background and rationale

Thoracic outlet syndrome may involve compression and/or stretching of the brachial plexus with subsequent neuropathic symptoms (Ide et al 2003). The subclavian artery and vein may also be compressed leading to vascular symptoms or deep vein thrombosis in the upper limb (Ofir & Eyal 2007). Thoracic outlet syndrome may be associated with postural changes or repetitive activities of the upper limb (Pascarelli & Hsu 2001). Shoulder bracing has been used by therapists to provide relief of symptoms by proposing to decrease the pressure or strain on the brachial plexus and subclavian artery and vein (Lyn Watson Shoulder Brace: http://www.sportstek.net/mslw.html [accessed 2 Oct 2009]). In the absence of a brace or an alternative to bracing, tape can be used to provide a mechanical lift to the arm and shoulder, thus decreasing the pressure or tension on the brachial plexus and/or subclavian artery and vein. This technique, if done effectively, should provide immediate relief from the upper limb neuropathic type symptoms and/or vascular symptoms. If moderate immediate relief of symptoms is not achieved, the technique should be reapplied or abandoned.

Evidence

○ No research studies relating to this technique were identified.

Material

○ Hypoallergenic underlay 3 × 20 cm strips.
○ Rigid tape 3 × 20 cm strips.

Patient position

○ Patient sits with feet well supported and pelvis in neutral position, the arm placed with shoulder in neutral position and elbow supported on 1–2 pillows.

Therapist position

○ Therapist stands beside the patient and assists the patient in positioning the scapula in the desired position.
○ Therapist gently elevates the GH joint by lifting the patient's arm upwards and towards the cervical spine.

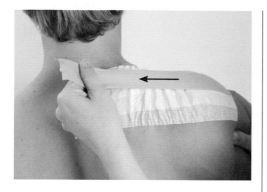

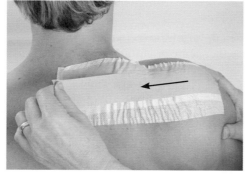

1 Apply hypoallergenic underlay starting on the superior and lateral aspect of the humerus. Lay the hypoallergenic underlay along the supraspinatus muscle finishing at the cervico-thoracic junction.

2 Repeat step 1 with a second strip of hypoallergenic underlay superimposing the first one by half.

3 Repeat step 2 with a third strip of hypoallergenic underlay superimposing the second one by half.

4 Apply the first strip of tape over the first strip of hypoallergenic underlay, starting at the superior and lateral aspect of the humerus. As you lay the tape over the supraspinatus muscle with one hand apply a superior lift of the humerus with the other hand. Finish the tape at the cervico-thoracic junction.

5 Repeat step 4 with the second and third strips of tape.

Reassessment
○ Upper limb, cervical and thoracic spine symptoms at rest.
○ Upper limb, cervical or thoracic spine provocative movements.

9

Shoulder joint

Overview
Although commonly used clinically and discussed in various texts in the literature, surprisingly few research studies relevant to the use of shoulder taping in either acute or chronic injury management, or in injury prevention, were identified. The techniques described have also varied greatly in their application, with some techniques using minimal tape with a couple of anchors and a few strips of tape around the shoulder while other techniques use an extensive amount of tape covering the entire shoulder. The techniques described in this section have specific therapeutic application and are based on physical examination findings.

Relocation of head of humerus (HOH) position

Background and rationale
In shoulder conditions the position of the HOH and its relevant movement in the glenoid has often been assessed by therapists as part of the routine shoulder physical examination. Altered HOH position as compared to the non-affected side has been thought to be a possible contributing cause to some shoulder symptoms (Hess 2000). The position of the HOH associated with functional instability may be difficult to diagnose and it could be anterior, posterior or inferior in relation to the glenoid (Guererro et al 2009).

For the following three techniques the HOH position and its relevant movement in the glenoid is assessed and compared to the non-affected side prior to the taping application. Relevant outcome measures are established for the presenting symptoms — for example, goniometric range of shoulder motion to first onset of pain (P1) — and pain level based on the visual analogue scale (VAS) or other numerical scales as discussed in Chapter 1. These measures can then be used post taping in evaluating the efficacy of the technique.

Evidence
- McConnell and McIntosh (2009) found that taping the HOH posteriorly (from an antero-superoposterior direction) increased ROM in internal, external and total rotation in male and female asymptomatic young tennis players (Level IV).
- Tape may be used to address humeral head position but published works are clinical or anecdotal reports (Hess 2000; McConnell 2000) (Clinical reports).

Antero-posterior relocation of HOH (antero-lateral taping)

Material
○ Hypoallergenic underlay 1 × 30 cm.
○ Rigid tape 1–2 × 30 cm strips.

Patient position
○ Patient sits with feet well supported and pelvis in neutral position.
○ Patient's arm is supported on a pillow in neutral shoulder position or in 30° abduction and neutral rotation.
○ Patient aims to actively set their scapulae in the position prescribed by the therapist.

Therapist position
○ Therapist stands beside the patient, facing shoulder to be taped.
○ Therapist further assists the scapulae in the prescribed position.

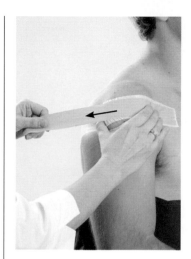

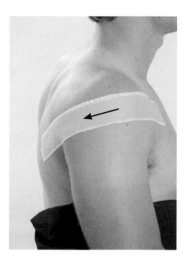

1 Apply the hypoallergenic underlay over the lateral aspect of the HOH, starting medial to the coracoid process and finishing inferior to the spine of the scapula.

2 Apply the tape over the underlay, starting anteriorly. Gently stabilise the scapula with one hand and relocate and glide HOH posteriorly into glenoid with the other hand.

3 Maintain the HOH posterior glide with one hand and tension the tape with the other hand. Place the tape posteriorly over the underlay while maintaining the tension but without pulling the tape so far as to compress into the skin.

4 Repeat step 3 if there is a need to reinforce the taping technique further. Often one strip of tape may suffice.

Reassessment
○ Position of HOH.
○ Symptomatic shoulder movement(s) and related symptoms.

Antero-posterior relocation of HOH (antero-superior taping)

Material
- Hypoallergenic underlay 1 × 30 cm.
- Rigid tape 1–2 × 30 cm strips.

Patient position
- Patient sits with feet well supported and pelvis in neutral position.
- Patient's arm is supported on a pillow in neutral shoulder position or in 30° abduction and neutral rotation.
- Patient aims to actively set their scapulae in the position prescribed by the therapist.

Therapist position
- Therapist stands beside the patient, facing shoulder to be taped.
- Therapist further assists the scapula into the prescribed position.

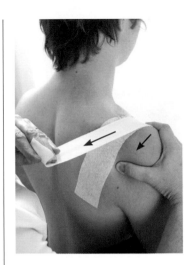

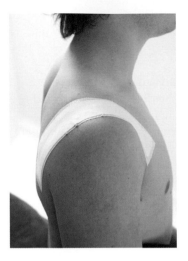

1 Apply the hypoallergenic underlay over the antero-superior aspect of the HOH, starting lateral to the coracoid process and anterior to the HOH, and finishing inferior to the spine of the scapula.
2 Apply the tape over the underlay, starting anteriorly. Gently stabilise the scapula with one hand and relocate and glide HOH posteriorly into glenoid with the other hand.

3 Maintain the HOH posterior glide with one hand and tension the tape with the other hand. Place the tape antero-superior and posteriorly over the underlay while maintaining the tension but without pulling the tape so far as to compress into the skin.
4 Repeat step 3 if there is a need to reinforce the taping technique further. Often one strip of tape may suffice.

Reassessment
- Position of HOH.
- Symptomatic shoulder movement(s) and related symptoms.

11

Relocation of HOH — postero-anterior (PA)

Material
- Hypoallergenic underlay 1 × 30 cm.
- Rigid tape 2 × 30 cm strips.

Patient position
- Patient sits with feet well supported and pelvis in neutral position.
- Patient's arm is supported on a pillow in neutral shoulder position or in 30° abduction and neutral rotation.
- Patient aims to actively set their scapulae in the position prescribed by the therapist.

Therapist position
- Therapist stands beside the patient, facing shoulder to be taped.
- Therapist further assists the scapula in the prescribed position.

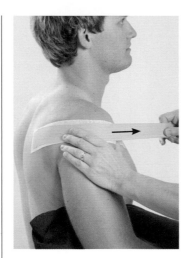

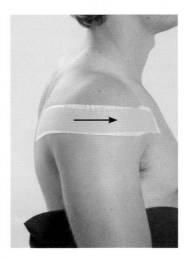

1 Apply the hypoallergenic underlay over the lateral aspect of the HOH, starting inferior to the spine of the scapula and finishing medial to the coracoid process.
2 Apply the tape over the underlay, starting posteriorly. Gently stabilise the scapula with one hand and relocate and glide HOH anteriorly into glenoid with the other hand.

3 Maintain the HOH anterior glide with one hand and tension tape with the other hand. Place anteriorly over the underlay while maintaining the tension but without pulling the tape so hard as to compress into the skin.
4 Repeat step 3 if there is a need to reinforce the taping technique further. Often one strip of tape may suffice.

Reassessment
- Position of HOH.
- Symptomatic shoulder movement(s) and related symptoms.

Relocation of HOH superiorly, for inferiorly subluxed HOH or multidirectional instability (MDI)

Background and rationale

The following taping technique can be used therapeutically for the GH joint. Indications for its use include patients with inferior instability, multidirectional instability or as part of the management of acute or chronic shoulder dislocation/ subluxation, both in the anterior or posterior directions. It is thought to provide mechanical support to the joint and neurophysiological proprioceptive input. It is still uncertain in the literature if this is the case though it is a clinically commonly used technique. Based on clinical observation, it has the added advantage of providing increased confidence to the patient, allowing them to move through their pain-free movement more confidently. It may also be used as an adjunct to shoulder bracing for shoulder multidirectional instability (Guererro et al 2009).

A similar technique to the one described here, but with added anterior and posterior oblique tape strips, is commonly used in injury prevention, such as dislocation or subluxation in contact or repetitive throwing sports. Whether the effects of the tape are mechanical, neurophysiological or merely psychological by increasing the confidence of the athletes is uncertain.

Material

○ Hypoallergenic underlay 2 × 20 cm strips.
○ Rigid tape 4 × 10 cm strips and 10 × 10 cm strips.

Patient position

○ Patient sits upright and comfortably on a chair, with the scapula set arm supported on a pillow in neutral position or in 30° abduction with neutral rotation.

Therapist position

○ Therapist stands beside the patient, on the side of the shoulder to be taped.

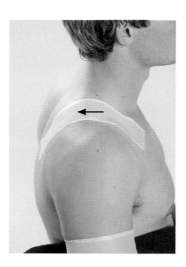

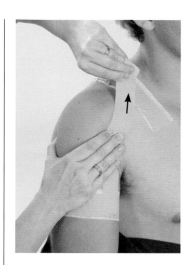

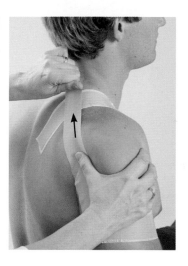

1 Apply two strips of hypoallergenic underlay, one strip over the clavicle starting medial to the coracoid process on the anterior aspect then directing the hypoallergenic underlay posteriorly over the spine of the scapula. The second strip is placed over the lateral aspect of the upper arm, approximately 2–3 cm below the deltoid insertion.

2 Apply tape anchors over the two strips of hypoallergenic underlay.

3 For inferior HOH position. Apply tape in a perpendicular direction starting on the inferior (upper arm) anchor and while relocating HOH superiorly with one hand, tension the tape and place onto the superior (clavicular) anchor with the other hand. Repeat 5–8 times, moving from the anterior to the posterior direction overlapping the previous strip of tape by half the width.

4 For inferior and posterior HOH position. Apply tape in a perpendicular direction starting posteriorly on the inferior (upper arm) anchor and while relocating HOH superiorly and anteriorly with one hand, tension the tape and place onto the superior (clavicular) anchor with the other hand. Repeat 5–8 times, moving from the posterior to anterior direction overlapping the previous strip of tape by half the width.

13

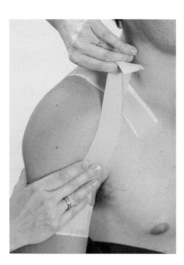

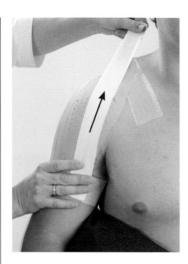

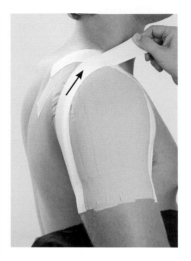

5 For inferior and anterior HOH position. Apply tape in a perpendicular direction starting anteriorly on the inferior (upper arm) anchor and while relocating HOH superiorly and also posteriorly with one hand. Tension the tape and place onto the superior (clavicular) anchor with the other hand. Repeat 5–8 times, moving from anterior to posterior direction overlapping the previous strip of tape by half the width.

6 If the taping is being performed on an athlete returning to sports post rehabilitation then two or more added strips of tape could be applied:

  6.1 apply a 15–20 cm tape strip anteriorly on the inferior anchor on the arm, lay it vertically in a superior direction until it passes anterior to the GH joint and then direct the tape obliquely over the AC joint to finish on the posterior aspect of the superior anchor

  6.2 apply a 15–20 cm tape strip posteriorly on the inferior anchor on the arm, lay it vertically in a superior direction until it passes posterior to the GH joint then direct the tape obliquely over the AC joint to finish on the anterior aspect of the superior anchor.

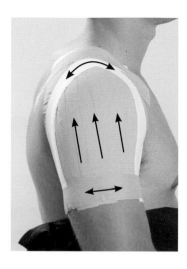

7 Apply two lock-offs over the anchors, one over the superior (clavicular) anchor and one over the inferior (upper arm) anchor.

Reassessment

○ Position of HOH.

○ Symptomatic movement or activity for symptom provocation.

○ Patient reported confidence with movement or activity.

Biceps tendon deloading technique

Background and rationale

In cases of biceps tendon pathology, using a technique to deload the biceps tendon may assist in temporarily decreasing pain and improving function.

Evidence

- No research studies relating to this taping technique were identified.
- Some research studies relating to the principle of using tape to deload or inhibit the injured tissues in other body regions such as the thoracic spine (O'Leary et al 2002) and lateral epicondylalgia of the elbow (Vicenzino et al 2003) have been published. The outcomes of these studies are described in a table in Appendix I.

Material

- Hypoallergenic underlay 2 × 5 cm strips and 1 × 20–25 cm strip.
- Rigid tape 2 × 20–25 cm strips and 4 × 3 cm strips.

Patient position

- Patient sits with feet well supported and pelvis in neutral position, arms placed by the side with shoulder in neutral position and forearm resting on a pillow in 30° elbow flexion and full forearm supination.

Therapist position

- Therapist stands beside the patient facing arm to be taped.

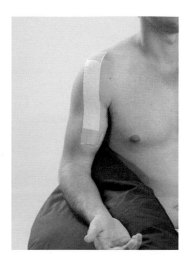 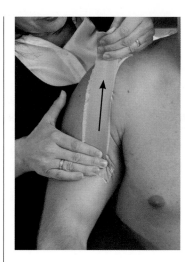 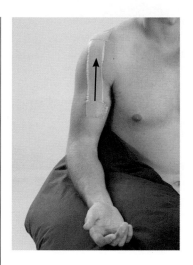

1 Apply one 5 cm strip of hypoallergenic underlay on the mid portion of the biceps belly (inferior anchor), and another 5 cm strip on the superior margin of the glenoid (superior anchor).

2 Apply the long strip of hypoallergenic underlay from the inferior to the superior anchor on the glenoid rim (near the origin of the long head of biceps tendon).

3 Apply the 2 × 5 cm rigid tape strips over the superior and inferior anchors of hypoallergenic underlay.

4 Apply a 20–25 cm rigid tape strip from the inferior anchor on the mid portion of the biceps belly and while gathering and lifting the biceps tendon upwards with one hand, tension the tape with the other hand and lay it down onto the superior glenoid rim anchor.

5 Repeat step 4 with a second 20–25 cm tape strip to reinforce the previous tape if required.

6 Repeat step 3, using another two 5 cm tape strips to lock-off the tape.

Reassessment
○ Symptomatic shoulder and elbow active ROM, and associated pain level.
○ Symptomatic functional tasks.

Shoulder external rotation limitation technique

Background and rationale

Excessive shoulder external rotation (ER) ROM may be concomitant to shoulder pathology (Burkhart & Lo 2007). It may thus be necessary in some patients to limit the amount of ER range of the shoulder in 90° of abduction. This can be achieved by the diagonal application of a long strip of tape used in this technique.

Evidence

○ No research studies relating to this technique were identified.

Material

○ Rigid tape 1 × 55–60 cm strip

Patient position

○ Patient is seated with the arm supported on a table or by the therapist in 90° abduction and in some internal rotation (IR).
○ The amount of IR rotation the shoulder is placed in for this taping technique will determine how much ER will be restricted. If the patient is placed in more IR starting position, the resultant ER will be less.

Therapist position

○ Therapist stands behind the patient, with the leg on a stool supporting the patient's arm position.

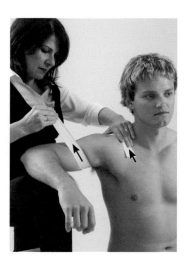

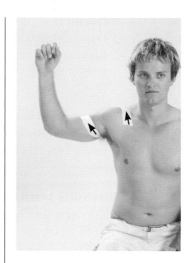

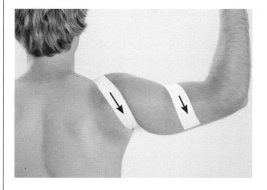

1 Start anteriorly, applying the tape over the pectoralis muscle group from below the coracoid process.

2 Direct the tape antero-posteriorly over the posterior GH joint line and inferiorly over the upper triceps brachii muscle.

3 Continue the tape anteriorly across the biceps brachii muscle and finish on the lateral aspect of the lower part of the upper arm.

4 The result should be a half spiral tape that limits external rotation of the GH joint.

Reassessment

○ Passive and active shoulder ER in 90° abduction. Ensure the desired amount of ER ROM is restricted.

15

Acromioclavicular joint

Background and rationale

The conservative management approach of mild acute or subacute acromioclavicular joint (ACJ) subluxation/dislocation usually includes some form of immobilisation through the use of slings or braces (Brukner & Khan 2007). Taping that provides support to the ACJ (Shamus & Shamus 1997; Stoddard & Johnson 2000) can be used as an adjunct to sling use in the acute phases and as an adjunct to manual therapy and exercise in the later stages of rehabilitation and return to activity. Brukner and Khan (2007) also describe the use of taping for the ACJ for return to sport.

Evidence

○ Shamus and Shamus (1997) described the use of ACJ taping in two case studies of ACJ injuries (Clinical report).
○ Stoddard and Johnson (2000) similarly advocate the use of a similar ACJ taping as an adjunct to treatment based on the outcome of a single case report (Clinical report).

Material

○ Hypoallergenic underlay 2 × 20–25 cm strips.
○ Rigid tape strips 4 × 20–25 cm for anchors and closing strips, and up to 10 × 20–25 cm strips, depending on the size of the patient.

Patient position

○ Patient sits upright and comfortably on a chair, arm supported on a pillow in neutral position or in 30° abduction with neutral rotation.

Therapist position

○ Therapist stands behind the patient, on the side of the shoulder to be taped.

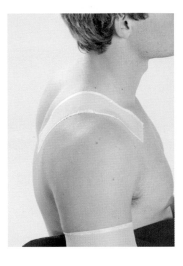

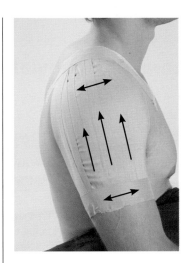

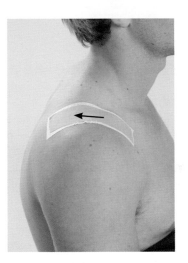

1 Apply two strips of hypoallergenic underlay:
   1.1 one strip over the proximal end of the clavicle starting lateral to the sternoclavicular joint anteriorly and direct tape posteriorly over the spine of the scapula
   1.2 one strip over the lateral aspect of the upper arm, approximately 2 cm below the deltoid insertion.
2 Apply tape anchors over the two strips of hypoallergenic underlay.

3 Apply a strip of tape in a perpendicular direction starting anteriorly on the inferior (upper arm) anchor and while lifting the distal end of humerus and acromion slightly upwards with one hand (to decrease the gravitational effect of the arm on the ACJ), tension the tape and place onto the superior (clavicular) anchor with the other hand. Repeat with additional strips of tape, moving from an anterior to posterior direction overlapping the previous strip of tape by half the width of the tape.
4 Apply lock-off strips over the anchors.
5 Follow points 6.1 and 6.2 from page 66.

6 For slight ACJ disruption or during the later stages of rehabilitation, 1–2 strips of tape over the ACJ may be sufficient to provide proprioceptive input to improve the pain and improve the ROM during the provocative movement.

Reassessment
○ Resting symptoms.
○ Provocative movements such as horizontal adduction, and associated symptoms.

Elbow joint

Elbow diamond deloading for lateral epicondylalgia

Background and rationale
Lateral epicondylalgia (LE) can be a functionally limiting condition with debilitating effects for the person experiencing it. Reducing strain on the common extensor tendon with a deloading technique has been shown to decrease pain and increase grip strength in a single blind randomised control study by Vicenzino et al (2003). This technique is based on that described by Vicenzino and colleagues (2003).

Evidence
O Vicenzino et al (2003) found that a diamond deloading taping technique decreased pain and increased grip strength in patients with LE (Level III-2).

Material
O Rigid tape $8 \times 8{-}10$ cm strips.
O Optional hypoallergenic underlay $4 \times 8{-}10$ cm strips.

Patient position
O Patient is supine with the forearm resting in slight flexion and pronation.
O Alternative position: patient is seated with arm resting on a pillow and elbow in slight flexion and pronation.

Therapist position
O Therapist stands beside the patient, facing the elbow to be taped.

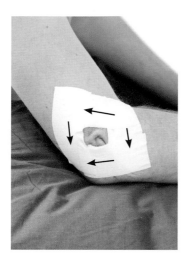

1 Apply the first strip of tape across the proximal end of the extensor muscles, gathering the tissues together at 90° to the direction of the tape.
2 Apply the second and subsequent strips of tape perpendicular to the previous strip to create a diamond shape around the common extensor tendon. As each piece of tape is laid down, gather the tissues towards the centre of the 'diamond box' ensuring the lateral epicondyle and common extensor origin remains in the centre of the 'box'.
3 Repeat with a second layer of four strips of tape gathering the tissues towards the centre of the diamond box as previously.
4 Hypoallergenic underlay can be applied underneath first if desired.

Reassessment
○ Pain free grip strength (using a handheld dynamometer)
○ Symptoms at rest and during provocative functional tasks.

17

Wrist extensor muscle deloading for lateral epicondylalgia

Background and rationale

In patients with lateral epicondylalgia (LE) the wrist extensor muscles may have increased activity and tightness. This taping technique may be used over the proximal extensor muscle bulk to deload or inhibit the overactive wrist extensor muscles. The subsequent effect may be reduction of pain and improvement in function during activation of the wrist extensor muscle group.

Evidence

○ No research studies relating to this technique were identified.

Material

○ Hypoallergenic underlay 1 × 5–10 cm strip.
○ Rigid tape 1 × 10 cm and 1 × 5–10 cm strips.

Patient position

○ Patient is supine with the forearm resting in slight flexion and pronation.

Therapist position

○ Therapist stands beside the patient.

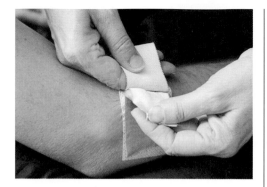

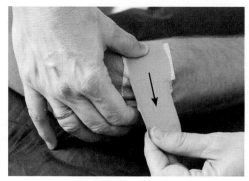

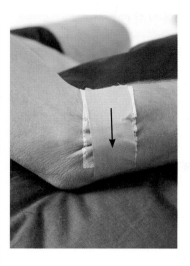

1   Apply hypoallergenic underlay perpendicular to the direction of the proximal muscle bulk of the wrist extensors.

2   Apply two pieces of tape, the medial one longer than the lateral, over the hypoallergenic underlay and pull and stick together the two pieces of tape.

3   Tension the tape holding it from the longer strip with one hand, while gathering the extensor muscle bulk in a perpendicular direction to the tape with the other hand.

4   Apply the tape from medial to lateral direction over the extensor muscles.

18

Reassessment

O   Pain free grip strength (using a handheld dynamometer).

O   Symptoms at rest and during provocative functional tasks.

Reinforcing elbow lateral glide for lateral epicondylalgia

Background and rationale

A manual therapy technique using an elbow lateral glide mobilisation with movement (MWM) technique has been advocated by Brian Mulligan to be effective in the treatment of lateral epicondylalgia (LE) (Mulligan 1999; Vicenzino & Wright 1995). This taping technique may be used to reinforce the MWM lateral glide of the elbow. Vicenzino and Wright (1995) included this taping technique as an adjunct to the treatment protocol of a patient with LE in a single case study. This technique utilises a spiral tape application to mimic the effects of the elbow lateral glide MWM technique. Once again, it is anticipated that this technique may lead to the reduction of pain and improvement in function.

Evidence

○ A single case study by Vicenzino and Wright (1995) found immediate improvement in pain-free grip strength in a patient with LE with the use of MWM lateral glide and taping together (Level IV).

Material

○ Rigid tape 1 × 40–50 cm strip.

Patient position

○ Patient is supine with the elbow supported in extension and the forearm in pronation.

Therapist position

○ Therapist stands beside the patient.

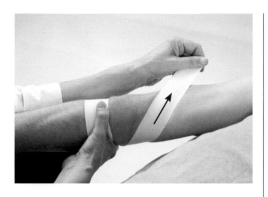

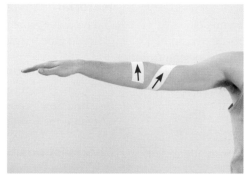

1   Apply the beginning of the tape on the postero-medial aspect of the forearm, immediately inferior to the elbow. Bring the tape anteriorly from medial to lateral, crossing the anterior aspect of the elbow joint.

2   Maintain the tension on the tape with one hand and apply a lateral glide on the elbow (this is where you wish you had more hands) with the other hand.

3   Bring the tape from the lateral elbow joint and fix it on the postero-lateral aspect of the distal humerus.

Reassessment
○ Pain-free grip strength (using a handheld dynamometer).
○ Symptoms at rest and during provocative functional tasks.

Limiting elbow extension

Background and rationale

After a traumatic injury to the elbow, one of the aims of rehabilitation may be to limit the amount of elbow extension range of motion. Tape can be used to limit the elbow motion to varying degrees of extension. The range limitation imposed on the elbow will depend on the injury and the pain-free available ROM, the patient's function and goals of treatment.

Evidence

- No research studies relating to this technique were identified.

Material

- Hypoallergenic underlay 2 × 20–30 cm strips.
- Rigid tape 4 × 20–30 cm and 4 × 20 cm strips.

Patient position

- Patient is supine with the forearm resting in supination.
- The elbow is positioned in the limit of extension range that the technique is intending to restrict.

Therapist position

- Therapist stands beside the patient.

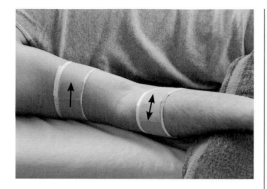 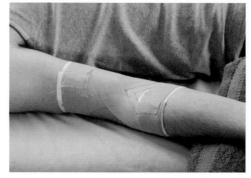

1 Apply hypoallergenic underlay for the proximal anchor around the humerus about 10 cm above the elbow and for the distal anchor, around the ulna and radius at about 10 cm below the elbow joint.

2 Apply two strips of 20–30 cm tape over the hypoallergenic underlay to act as anchors.

3 Apply a single 20 cm strip of tape in an oblique direction starting on the anterior aspect of the elbow, from the medial aspect of the distal anchor to lateral aspect of the proximal anchor.

4 Apply a single 20 cm strip of tape from the lateral aspect of the distal anchor to the medial aspect of the proximal anchor in an oblique direction while maintaining the tension on the tape. The two strips of tape should form an X.

5 Repeat steps 3 and 4, overlapping the previous two strips of tape with a second layer.

6 Repeat step 2, using two 20–30 cm strips of tape over the original anchors, with the tape application to act as lock-offs.

Reassessment

○ Symptoms at rest and during movement.

○ Elbow extension range of motion.

20

Limiting elbow valgus motion

Background and rationale

Elbow valgus motion may result from excessive ulnar collateral ligament laxity caused by a traumatic injury or from repetitive strain such as occurs in throwers (Andrews et al 1993). Tape applied medially on the elbow in a criss-cross direction that prevents excessive valgus motion may prevent further injury and pain.

Evidence

○ No research studies relating to this technique were identified.

Material

○ Hypoallergenic underlay 2 × 20–30 cm strips.
○ Rigid tape 4 × 20–30 cm and 4 × 15 cm strips.

Patient position

○ Patient is supine with the forearm resting in supination and 15–20° flexion, in the position to be taped.
○ This technique can also be done with the patient seated.

Therapist position

○ Therapist stands beside the patient.

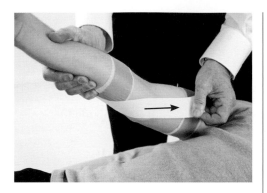 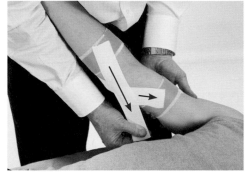 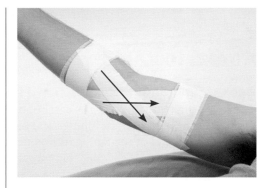

1 Apply hypoallergenic underlay around the humerus for the proximal anchor, about 10 cm above the elbow and around the ulna and radius for the distal anchor at about 10 cm below the elbow joint.

2 Apply the two strips of 20–30 cm tape over the hypoallergenic underlay to act as anchors.

3 Apply a single 15 cm strip of tape from the distal to the proximal anchor on the medial side of the elbow while maintaining the tension on the tape, directing the tape from medial to lateral in an oblique direction.

4 Apply a single 15 cm strip of tape from the distal to the proximal anchor on the medial side of the elbow while maintaining the tension on the tape, directing the tape from lateral to medial in an oblique direction. The two strips of tape should form an X.

5 Repeat steps 3 and 4, overlapping each previous strip of tape by half with a second layer of tape.

6 Apply two 20–30 cm strips of tape over the anchors to act as lock-offs over the tape.

Reassessment
○ Passive elbow valgus motion.
○ Symptoms at rest and during movement.
○ Functional tasks.

Carpal instability

Background and rationale
The following taping techniques can be adapted and used as part of the management of wrist injuries and particularly in cases of carpal instability. For the taping techniques to be effective, accurate assessment of the unstable carpal involved is essential. The involved carpals are identified using specific carpal stress tests (Young et al 2007) and accessory glides (Staes et al 2009). Some of the most commonly identified carpals involved in wrist instability are the scaphoid and/or lunate in scaphoid–lunate dissociation and the triquetrum in triangular fibrocartilaginous complex (TFCC) injuries. Once the involved carpals are identified the taping techniques will be guided by which carpal accessory movement relieves the patient's symptoms of pain and/or increases the pain-free wrist motion or functional tasks. The taping is applied around the wrist after the carpal glide has been performed. Often it may be more effective to form a small foam buttress, placed over the relevant carpal and under the tape to further enhance the glide (Prosser 1995).

Evidence
- No research studies relating to this technique were identified.
- A similar technique was described for TFCC injuries by Prosser (1995) in a clinical case report (Clinical report).

Material
- Hypoallergenic underlay 1 × 20–25 cm strip (optional).
- Rigid tape 1 × 20–25 cm strip.

Patient position
- Patient is supine with the forearm supported in pronation and the wrist in neutral position.
- This technique can also be done with the patient seated.

Therapist position
- Therapist stands beside the patient.

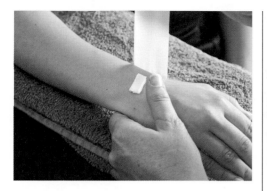

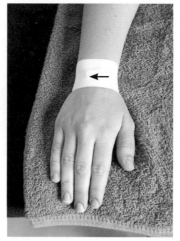

1 Apply hypoallergenic underlay around the wrist if preferred.
2 Place the start of the tape on the dorsum or palmar aspect of the wrist.
3 Once the specific carpal bone to be stabilised and the direction of the required glide to reduce symptoms (palmar or dorsal) has been identified, the glide is applied with one hand while the tape is tensioned with the other hand and placed around the wrist.

4 The two ends of the tape are overlapped in slight oblique direction.
5 If a carpal buttress is used, it needs to be placed over the carpal side where the glide is applied from (palmar side for a dorsal glide and on the dorsal side for a palmar glide).

Reassessment
○ Symptoms at rest.
○ Provocative wrist ROM movement, provocative task and symptoms.

22

Ulnar carpal instability

Background and rationale

The following taping technique more specifically addresses instability of the ulnar carpus (ulna, lunate and triquetrum), with involvement of the TFCC. Often a traumatic injury of TFCC may involve the ulnar collateral ligament and the distal radioulnar joint (Prosser 1995) which can lead to increased laxity on the ulnar aspect of the wrist. Taping can be used as in the previous technique, however, it will need to commence on the palmar aspect of the wrist and then be directed medially to the dorsal aspect in order to lift the involved triquetrum and approximate it to the ulna and the lunate during the taping procedure.

Evidence

○ No research studies relating to this technique were identified.
○ A similar technique to the one described here was used in a single case report as part of the conservative management of ulnar carpal instability by Prosser (1995) (Clinical report).

Material

○ Hypoallergenic underlay 1 × 20–25 cm strip (optional).
○ Rigid tape 1 × 20–25 cm strip.

Patient position

○ Patient is supine with the forearm supported in pronation and the wrist in neutral position.
○ This technique can also be done with the patient seated.

Therapist position

○ Therapist stands beside the patient.

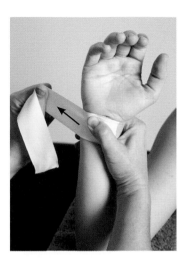
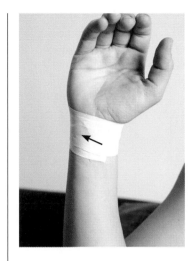

1 Apply hypoallergenic underlay around the wrist if preferred.

2 Place the start of the tape on the palmar aspect of the wrist, starting from the radial side towards the ulnar side.

3 A passive accessory glide is applied on the triquetrum in a dorsal direction with one hand. The tape is tensioned with the other hand and placed around the wrist from the ulnar side towards the radial side and finishing on the dorsal aspect.

4 The two ends of the tape are overlapped in slight oblique direction.

5 If a carpal buttress is used, it needs to be placed on the palmar aspect of the triquetrum prior to applying the passive accessory dorsal glide and completing the taping technique.

Reassessment
○ Symptoms at rest.
○ Provocative wrist ROM movement, functional task and symptoms.

Wrist extension ROM limitation

Background and rationale

This technique aims to limit the range of wrist motion into extension. Clinical indications include cases where wrist extension is pain provocative or hyper-mobile. The technique incorporates a criss-cross tape effect and it is similar for both the limitation of flexion and extension techniques. Using this technique as part of the therapy management of patients who require long-term wrist support is useful in the interim period until a suitable wrist brace or splint is obtained.

Evidence

○ No research studies relating to this technique were identified.

Material

○ Hypoallergenic underlay 2 × 20–25 cm strips.
○ Rigid tape 4 × 20–25 cm strips.
○ Rigid tape 4 × 15–20 cm strips.

Patient position

○ Patient is seated with the forearm in neutral position, the elbow flexed to 90° resting on a table.
○ Wrist is positioned in flexion (amount of flexion position will depend on the desired extension limitation).

Therapist position

○ Therapist stands or sits facing the patient's wrist and hand.

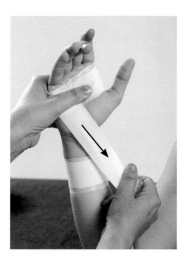

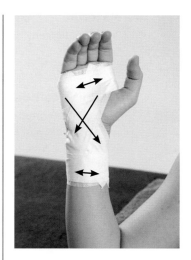

1 Apply hypoallergenic underlay for the proximal anchor 5 cm above the radial and ulnar styloid processes.

2 Apply hypoallergenic underlay for the distal anchor around the palm, over the second to fifth metacarpals.

3 Apply a single 20–25 cm strip of tape as a proximal anchor over the hypoallergenic underlay, 5 cm above the carpus.

4 Apply a single 20–25 cm strip of tape as a distal anchor over the hypoallergenic underlay around the palm, over the distal second to fifth metacarpals.

5 Apply a tensioned 15–20 cm strip of tape on the palmar aspect of the wrist from the ulnar side of the distal anchor to the radial side of the proximal anchor, in an oblique direction.

6 Apply a tensioned 15–20 cm strip of tape on the palmar aspect of the hand from the radial side of the distal anchor to the ulnar side of the proximal anchor, forming an X.

7 Repeat steps 5 and 6 with a second layer overlapping the tape by half its width.

8 Apply two 20–25 cm strips of tape as lock-offs, over the superior and the inferior anchors.

Reassessment

○ Passive and active wrist extension ROM
○ Provocative functional task and symptoms.

Wrist flexion ROM limitation

Background and rationale

This technique aims to limit the range of wrist motion into flexion. It is clinically indicated in cases where wrist flexion is pain provocative or hyper-mobile. The technique incorporates a criss-cross tape effect and it is similar for the limitation of both flexion and extension. This technique is useful in the interim period of management of patients who require long-term wrist support, until a suitable wrist brace or splint is obtained.

Evidence

○ No research studies relating to this technique were identified.

Material

○ Hypoallergenic underlay 2 × 20–25 cm strips.
○ Rigid tape 4 × 20–25 cm strips.
○ Rigid tape 4 × 15–20 cm strips.

Patient position

○ Patient is seated with the forearm in neutral position, the elbow flexed to 90° resting on a table.
○ The wrist is held in a degree of extension relevant to the amount of flexion limitation that is required.

Therapist position

○ Therapist stands or sits facing the patient's wrist and hand.

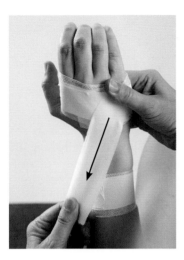

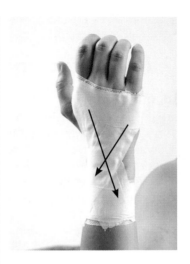

25

1   Apply hypoallergenic underlay for the proximal anchor 5 cm above the radial and ulnar styloid processes.
2   Apply hypoallergenic underlay for the distal anchor around the palm, over the second to fifth metacarpals.
3   Apply a single 20–25 cm strip of tape as a proximal anchor over the hypoallergenic underlay, 5 cm above the carpus.
4   Apply a single 20–25 cm strip of tape as a distal anchor over the hypoallergenic underlay around the palm, over the distal second to fifth metacarpals.
5   Apply a tensioned 15–20 cm strip of tape on the dorsal aspect of the hand from the ulnar side of the distal anchor to the radial side of the proximal anchor.
6   Apply a tensioned 15–20 cm strip of tape on the dorsal aspect of the hand from the radial side of the distal anchor to the ulnar side of the proximal anchor, forming a criss-cross.

7   Repeat steps 5 and 6, overlapping the tape by half its width.
8   Apply two 20–25 cm strips of tape as lock-offs, over the superior and the inferior anchors.

Reassessment

○ Passive and active wrist flexion ROM.
○ Provocative functional task and symptoms.

Hand, thumb and finger

Thumb carpometacarpal thumb spica

Background and rationale

Carpometacarpal (CMC) osteoarthritis (OA) of the thumb is a common condition, especially in older adults (Cook & Lalonde 2008). The following taping technique is used to provide mechanical support to the CMC joint during the inflammatory phase, while allowing the interphalangeal and/or the metacarpophalangeal joints to move. Taping can also be used in the interim period until a suitable brace or splint is obtained which may provide better long-term support and symptom relief for the patient (Cook & Lalonde 2008). This technique is also useful for other CMC injuries.

Evidence

- No research studies relating to this technique were identified.
- Timm (1985) described a thumb spica taping technique for first metacarpophalangeal (MCP) joint strains (Clinical report).

Material

- Hypoallergenic underlay 1 × 20–25 cm strip (optional).
- Rigid tape 2 × 20–25 cm strips.
- Rigid tape 8–10 × 15–20 cm strips torn longitudinally in half (19 mm width).

Patient position

- Patient is seated with the forearm in neutral position, elbow flexed and resting on a table.
- The wrist is held in the functional position and the thumb is abducted.

Therapist position

- Therapist stands or sits facing the patient's wrist and hand.

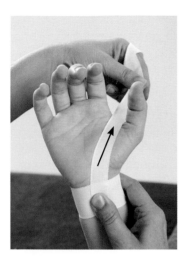

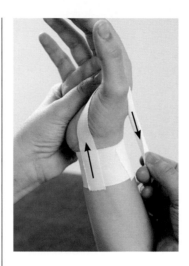

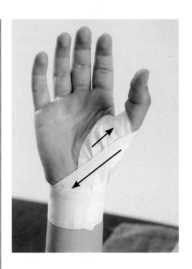

26

1 Apply hypoallergenic underlay around the wrist, above the ulnar and radial styloids (optional).
2 Apply one 20–25 cm strip of tape over the hypoallergenic underlay, to act as an anchor around the wrist.
3 Attach one 19 mm tape strip on the anchor on the palmar side of the thumb medial to the radius.
4 Tension the tape and lay it over the web space, directing the tape dorsally towards the wrist and back onto the anchor on the dorsal aspect.

5 Repeat step 3 several times, as required by the size of the patient's wrist and hand, each time overlapping the tape by half its width and moving the overlapped tape from the ulnar to the radial aspect of the thenar eminence.

6 Apply one rigid 20–25 cm strip of tape as a lock-off around the wrist to secure the spica strips of tape in place.

Reassessment
○ Symptoms at rest.
○ Passive and active thumb ROM, especially CMC.
○ Provocative thumb movements, functional tasks and symptoms.

Thumb ulnar collateral ligament injury

Background and rationale

Trauma to the ulnar collateral ligament of the thumb commonly occurs in sports (Folk 2001). The following taping technique can be used in acute or subacute injuries and during the rehabilitation phase. It can also be used in the interim period until a suitable brace or splint is obtained to provide better long-term support and symptom relief for the patient. The aim of the technique is to provide mechanical support to the metacarpophalangeal (MCP) joint while allowing the interphalangeal joint to move.

Evidence

- No research studies relating to this technique were identified.
- Timm (1985) described a thumb spica taping technique for first MCP joint strains (Clinical report).

Material

- Hypoallergenic underlay 1 × 20–25 cm strip (optional).
- Rigid tape 2 × 20–25 cm strips.
- Rigid tape 5 × 25–30 cm strips torn longitudinally in half (19 mm width).

Patient position

- Patient is seated with the forearm in neutral position, elbow flexed and resting on a table.
- The wrist is held in the functional position and the MCP joint of the thumb is in 30° flexion.

Therapist position

- Therapist stands or sits facing the patient's wrist and hand.

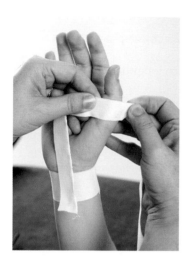 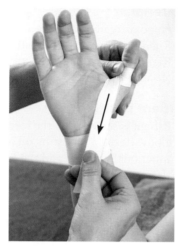 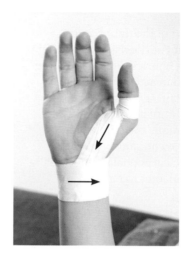 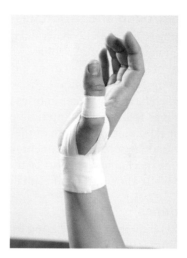

1 Apply hypoallergenic underlay around the wrist, at the ulnar and radial styloids (optional).

2 Apply one 20–25 cm strip of tape over the hypoallergenic underlay, to act as an anchor around the wrist.

3 Place the centre of a 19 mm tape strip on the lateral aspect of the proximal phalanx of the thumb.

4 Tension the medial end of the 19 mm tape strip, cross it and place it over the web space directed towards the dorsal inferior radioulnar joint.

5 Tension the lateral end of the 19 mm tape strip and place it over the web space so the tape crosses over the medial aspect of the thumb MCP and is directed towards the palmar inferior radioulnar joint.

6 Repeat steps 4 to 6 up to 2–3 times, each time overlapping the tape by half its width and moving the overlapped tape from medial to lateral aspect of the thenar eminence.

7 Apply one rigid 20–25 cm strip of tape as a lock-off around the wrist to secure the spica strips of tape in place.

Reassessment

○ Symptoms at rest.
○ Passive valgus test at the MCP joint.
○ Passive and active thumb ROM, especially MCP flexion and extension.
○ Provocative thumb movements, functional tasks and symptoms.

Thumb radial collateral ligament injury

Background and rationale
Trauma to the radial collateral ligament of the thumb is less common than the ulnar collateral ligament (Edelstein et al 2008) but nonetheless does occur in sporting injuries (Folk 2001). The following taping technique can be used in acute or subacute radial collateral ligament injuries and during the rehabilitation phases as well as in the interim period until a suitable brace or splint is obtained. The aim of the technique is similar to the thumb ulnar collateral ligament injury technique, namely to provide mechanical support to the metacarpophalangeal (MCP) joint while allowing the interphalangeal joint to move.

Evidence
- No research studies relating to this technique were identified.
- Timm (1985) described a thumb spica taping technique for first MCP joint strains (Clinical report).

Material
- Hypoallergenic underlay 1 × 20–25 cm strip (optional).
- Rigid tape 2 × 20–25 cm strips.
- Rigid tape 5 × 25–30 cm strips torn longitudinally in half (19 mm width).

Patient position
- Patient is seated with the forearm in neutral position with the elbow flexed and resting on a table. The wrist is held in the functional position and the MCP joint of the thumb is in 30° flexion.

Therapist position
- Therapist stands or sits facing the patient's wrist and hand.

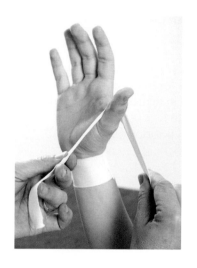 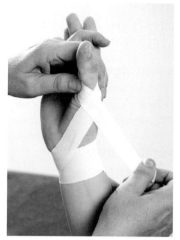 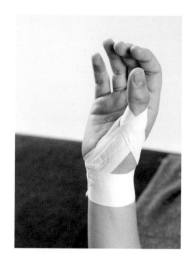 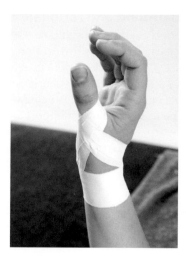

28

1 Apply hypoallergenic underlay around the wrist, at the ulnar and radial styloids (optional).

2 Apply one 20–25 cm strip of tape over the hypoallergenic underlay, to act as an anchor around the wrist.

3 Place the centre of a 19 mm tape strip on the medial aspect of the proximal phalanx of the thumb.

4 Tension the medial end of the 19 mm strip of tape and bring it over the thenar eminence and around the thumb, directed towards the dorsal inferior radioulnar joint.

5 Tension the lateral end of the 19 mm strip of tape and bring it around the thumb so the tape crosses over the lateral aspect of the thumb MCP and is directed towards the palmar side of the inferior radioulnar joint.

6 Repeat steps 4 and 5 up to 2–3 times, each time overlapping the tape by half its width and moving the overlapped tape from medial to lateral aspect of the thenar eminence.

7 Apply one rigid 20–25 cm strip of tape as a lock-off around the wrist to secure the spica strips of tape in place.

Reassessment

○ Symptoms at rest.
○ Passive varus test at the MCP joint.
○ Passive and active thumb ROM, especially MC flexion and extension.
○ Provocative thumb movements, functional tasks and symptoms.

Metacarpal fractures

Background and rationale

Part of the conservative management of non-displaced stable metacarpal fractures involves protective immobilisation for a period of 4–6 weeks before progressing to the use of splints (Hardy 2004). As the patient is rehabilitating and returning to sports or function, and is being weaned from the splint, taping can be used to provide support and proprioceptive input to the metacarpals. This taping technique can be performed using either rigid tape or elasticised tape, depending on the availability of the elasticised tape and the degree of support desired.

Evidence

Poolman et al (2005) conducted a Cochrane systematic review on conservative management options for closed fractures of the fifth metacarpal that included taping as a treatment option. They concluded that no conservative treatment option was superior to the others that had been studied, and also that recovery was excellent regardless of the conservative treatment used (Level I).

Material

○ Rigid tape 1 × 20–25 cm strip.
○ Alternatively, use elasticised tape.

Patient position

○ Patient is seated with the forearm in neutral position with the elbow flexed and resting on a table.
○ The wrist is held in the functional position.

Therapist position

○ Therapist stands or sits facing the patient's wrist and hand.

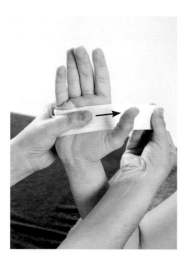

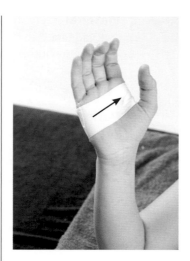

1 Attach one end of the 20–25 cm strip of tape on the dorsum of the hand at the 3rd metacarpal directing the tape towards the ulnar side.

2 Tension the tape and bring it towards the fifth metacarpal around the ulnar aspect of the hand in a slight oblique direction, over the palm of the hand, applying it between the web space and over to meet the other end in an oblique direction.

3 Care must be taken not to compress the metacarpals together and to avoid any skin folds while taping as this can be very uncomfortable for the patient.

Reassessment
○ Symptoms at rest.
○ Provocative hand movements, functional tasks and symptoms.

29

Finger buddy taping

Background and rationale

Finger buddy taping is often used in sport for on-field management of finger injuries, especially for interphalangeal (IP) second to fifth finger injuries. It is a useful technique for immobilising an affected digit using the neighbouring non-affected digit. It is equally useful when a patient is returning to sports or functional activity after a finger injury and the aim of the treatment is to provide support to the injured digit (Singletary et al 2003). Various buddy taping techniques are used, perhaps most commonly utilising two small strips of tape, one around each of the phalanges adjacent to the injured IP joint. The variation of the buddy taping technique described in this section uses a figure-of-8 taping method and it can be applied to allow flexion at the proximal IP joints and immobilising the distal IP joints, or alternatively to limit motion at both the proximal IP joints and the distal IP joints. For instance, if it is used to support a volar plate fracture when splinting is not available or when splinting use is being decreased, then both the distal and proximal IP joints will be immobilised into extension using the buddy taping technique (Yamazaki et al 2005).

It is important to note that tape used in the management of acute finger injuries needs to be applied in conjunction with management of acute oedema and pain. If a cohesive tape is used to manage the finger swelling, the taping technique described here can be performed over the cohesive tape.

Evidence

○ No research studies relating to this technique were identified.

Material

○ Rigid tape 2 × 10–15 cm strips torn longitudinally in half (19 mm width).
○ Alternatively 2 × 10–15 cm strips elasticised tape (19 mm width).

Patient position

○ Patient is seated with the forearm in neutral position, elbow flexed and resting on a table.
○ The wrist is held in the functional position and the metacarpophalangeal (MCP) joints of the fingers in slight flexion.

Therapist position

○ Therapist stands or sits facing the patient's wrist and hand.

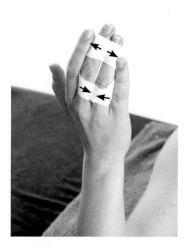

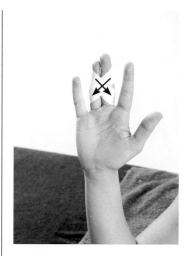

Procedure A: to allow flexion at the proximal IP joints

1 Place a soft pad between the two fingers to be taped to ensure more comfort for the patient. If there is no material to provide a pad such as a high-density foam, fold a small piece of tape together into three or four layers and place it between the two fingers.
2 Attach one end of the 19 mm strip of tape horizontally on the dorsum of the middle phalanx of the first finger to be immobilised (buddy taped) and bring tape horizontally towards the palmar aspect.

3 Bring tape obliquely over the palmar aspect of the proximal IP joints and finish the tape on the dorsum of the proximal phalanx of the first finger to be immobilised.
4 Apply one end of the second 19 mm strip of tape horizontally on the dorsum of the middle phalanx of the fingers to be immobilised, in the opposite direction of the tape in step 2 (i.e. direct one strip of tape towards the radial and one strip of tape towards the ulnar aspects).
5 Bring tape obliquely over the proximal IP joints and finish on the proximal phalanx of the first finger to be immobilised.
6 The two strips of tape should form an X taping effect on the palmar aspect of the proximal IP joints. This should allow the proximal IP joints to flex together.

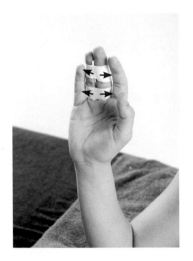

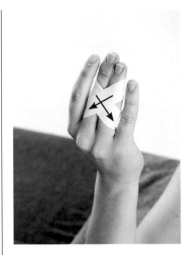

30

Procedure B: to limit flexion at the proximal IP joints

1 Place a soft pad between the two fingers to be taped to ensure more comfort for the patient. If there is no material to provide a pad, fold a small piece of tape together into three or four layers and place it between the two fingers.
2 Attach one end of the 19 mm strip of tape horizontally on the palmar aspect of the middle phalanx of one of the fingers to be immobilised.

3 Bring tape obliquely over the dorsal aspect of the proximal IP joints and finish tape on the palmar aspect of the proximal phalanx of the first finger to be immobilised.
4 Apply one end of the second 19 mm strip of tape horizontally on the palmar aspect of the middle phalanx of the second finger to be immobilised in the opposite direction of the tape in step 2 (i.e. direct one strip of tape toward the radial aspect and the other strip toward the ulnar aspect).
5 Bring tape obliquely over the dorsal aspect of the proximal IP joints and finish tape on the proximal phalanx of the first finger to be immobilised.
6 The 2 strips of tape should form an X taping effect on the dorsal aspect of the proximal IP joints, stabilising the fingers in extension.

Reassessment

○ Circulation, patient comfort and symptoms at rest.
○ MCP or IP joints passive and active ROM controlled by taping.

'Mallet finger' — flexion deformity of the distal interphalangeal joint

Background and rationale

The commonly used term 'mallet finger' refers to a flexion deformity of the distal interphalangeal (DIP) joint which involves a disruption of the terminal extensor tendon (Kovacic et al 2005). The injury may also involve an avulsion fracture at the site of the tendon insertion at the base of the distal phalanx. The initial management of tendon avulsion without fractures or with small non-displaced fractures is preferably conservative and involves immobilisation of the DIP joint for up to 6 weeks using a splint (Bendre et al 2005; Tuttle et al 2006) and gradually removing the splint for longer periods during the day, only wearing it at night (Singletary et al 2003) for a further 4–6 weeks, to allow the patient to commence functional activity. This taping technique, which utilises a figure-of-8 application, can be used to support the DIP joint during the period when the patient is being weaned from the continuous splint use.

Taping may also be used to manage the initial DIP sporting injury, immobilising the finger until further assessment and radiological examination is undertaken to exclude fractures. As discussed previously, taping is only an adjunct to other modalities in managing acute finger injuries with oedema and pain.

Evidence

○ No research studies relating to this technique were identified.

Material

○ Rigid tape 1 × 10 cm strip torn longitudinally in half (19 mm width) resulting in 2 × 10 cm × 19 mm tape strips.
○ Alternatively 2 × 10 cm strip elasticised narrow tape (19 mm width).

Patient position

○ Patient is seated with the forearm in neutral position, elbow flexed and resting on a table.
○ The wrist is held in the functional position, the metacarpophalangeal (MCP) joints in slight flexion and the fingers in extension.

Therapist position

○ Therapist stands or sits facing the patient's wrist and hand.

31

31

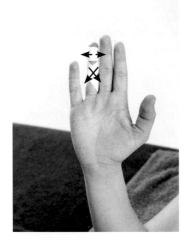

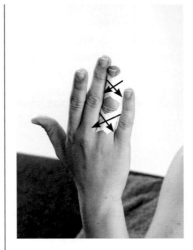

1 Attach one end of the 19 mm strip of tape on the palmar aspect of the distal phalanx.

2 Tension the tape and apply either medially or laterally towards the dorsal aspect crossing obliquely over the dorsal DIP joint and continuing the tape in a spiral direction over the palmar aspect of the middle phalanx to finish on the dorsal aspect of the proximal phalanx.

3 Repeat step 2 applying tape in the opposite direction.

4 Finish the tape on the dorsal aspect of the proximal phalanx overlapping it over the end of the first strip of tape.

Reassessment

○ Circulation, patient comfort and symptoms at rest.

○ Passive and active restriction of ROM of DIP flexion.

○ Provocative movement of the finger and symptoms.

'Jersey finger' — hyperextension deformity of the distal interphalangeal joint

Background and rationale

'Jersey finger' commonly refers to the hyperextension deformity of the distal interphalangeal (DIP) joint resulting from an injury to the flexor digitorum profundus. The injury is usually classified into Type I–V, depending on the retraction of the tendon stump and the presence of an avulsion fracture or a fracture of the distal phalanx (Tuttle et al 2006; Shippert 2007). The injury is usually managed surgically with reattachment of the tendon and internal fixation of the fracture (Tuttle et al 2006). Postoperative management varies with early mobilisation preferred by some surgeons (Shabat et al 2002) and splinting with controlled mobilisation by others (Kovacic et al 2005).

Taping can be used during the mobilisation or controlled mobilisation period to allow normal flexion motion and prevent hyperextension at the DIP joint. Similarly to mallet finger, taping may also be used to manage the acute injury to immobilise the DIP joint until the patient can be examined by a physician to ascertain the extent of the injury.

Evidence

○ No research studies relating to this technique were identified.

Material

○ Rigid tape 1 × 10 cm strip torn longitudinally in half (19 mm width) resulting in 2 × 10 cm × 19 mm tape strips.
○ Alternatively 2 × 10 cm strip elasticised tape (19 mm width).

Patient position

○ Patient is seated with the forearm in neutral position, elbow flexed and resting on a table.
○ The wrist is held in the functional position, the metacarpophalangeal (MCP) joints in slight flexion and the fingers in extension.

Therapist position

○ Therapist stands or sits facing the patient's wrist and hand.

32

32

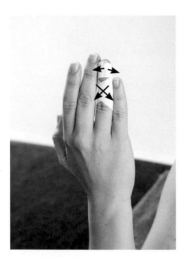

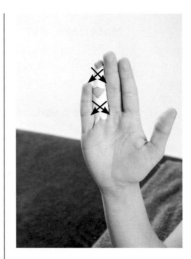

1 Attach one end of the 19 mm strip of tape on the dorsal aspect of the distal phalanx.
2 Tension the tape and apply either medially or laterally towards the palmar aspect crossing obliquely over the palmar DIP joint and continuing the tape in a spiral direction over the dorsal aspect of the middle phalanx to finish on the palmar proximal phalanx.

3 Repeat step 2 applying tape in the opposite direction.
4 Finish the tape on the palmar aspect of the proximal phalanx overlapping it over the end of the first strip of tape.

Reassessment
○ Circulation, patient comfort and symptoms at rest.
○ Passive and active restriction of ROM of DIP extension.
○ Provocative movement of the finger and symptoms.

Finger Boutonniere Deformity — flexion deformity of the proximal interphalangeal joint and hyperextension deformity at the distal interphalangeal joint

Background and rationale

'Boutonniere Deformity' is another commonly used term in finger injuries which refers to a flexion deformity of the proximal interphalangeal (PIP) joint and a hyperextension deformity at the distal interphalangeal (DIP) joint from traumatic loss of the extensor mechanism at the PIP joint (Coons & Green 1995). Usual management of the tendon disruption involves splinting of the PIP joint in full extension for 6–8 weeks, whereas surgical repair is recommended for more extensive injury, which may also involve avulsion fracture or fracture of the phalanx (Peterson et al 2006).

Taping can be applied to support the PIP joint in extension as interim management of an acute injury, until the patient is able to be further assessed and managed by a physician. Similarly, as in previous techniques, taping can be used as the patient is being weaned from the splint.

Evidence

○ No research studies relating to this technique were identified.

Material

○ Rigid tape 1 × 10 cm strip torn longitudinally in half (19 mm width) resulting in 2 × 10 cm × 19 mm tape strips.
○ Alternatively, use 2 × 10 cm strips elasticised tape (19 mm width).

Patient position

○ Patient is seated with the forearm in neutral position, elbow flexed and resting on a table.
○ The wrist is held in the functional position, the metacarpophalangeal (MCP) joints in slight flexion and the fingers in extension.

Therapist position

○ Therapist stands or sits facing the patient's wrist and hand.

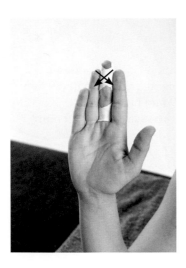 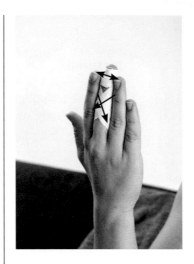

33

1 Attach one end of the 19 mm strip of tape on the dorsal aspect of the distal phalanx.
2 Tension the tape and apply either medially or laterally towards the palmar aspect crossing obliquely over the palmar DIP joint and continuing the tape in a spiral direction crossing obliquely over the dorsal PIP joint to finish on the palmar aspect of the proximal phalanx.

3 Repeat step 2, applying tape in the opposite direction.
4 Finish the tape on the palmar aspect of the proximal phalanx overlapping it over the end of the first strip of tape.

Reassessment
○ Circulation, patient comfort and symptoms at rest.
○ Passive and active restriction of ROM of DIP extension and PIP flexion.
○ Provocative movement of the finger and symptoms.

Finger rotation or translation positional malalignment of the phalanges

Background and rationale

Traumatic injuries to the fingers may often include disruption to the volar plate, the extensor mechanism of the phalanges, the ulnar or medial collateral ligaments, fractures, dislocations or combinations of these. Even after the initial symptoms have subsided, and the initial injury healed, patients may still be experiencing pain and stiffness or loss of ROM with certain movements or tasks. Clinical findings may reveal rotation or translation positional malalignment of the phalanges in relation to each other. Either rigid or elastic narrow (19 mm) tape can be used to support the phalanges in the position that relieves or least provokes patients' symptoms, while possibly correcting the positional malalignment. This technique is based on Brian Mulligan's principles of mobilisation with movement (MWM) (Mulligan 1999). The technique involves a spiral application of tape on the involved phalanx.

Evidence

○ No research studies relating to this technique were identified.

Material

○ Rigid tape 1 × 15 cm strip torn longitudinally in half (19 mm width).
○ Alternatively 1 × 15 cm strip elasticised tape (19 mm width).

Patient position

○ Patient is seated with the forearm in neutral position, elbow flexed and resting on a table.
○ The wrist is held in the functional position, the metacarpophalangeal (MCP) joints in slight flexion and the fingers in extension.

Therapist position

○ The therapist stands or sits facing the patient's wrist and hand.

34

34

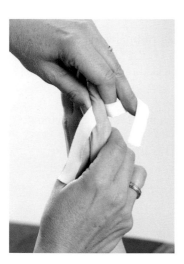

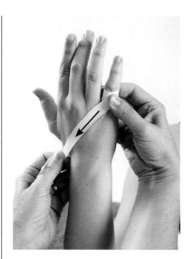

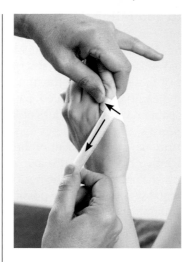

1 Identify the provocative movement of the involved interphalangeal joint in flexion or extension.
2 Identify the involved phalanx and the direction of positional malalignment, either medial or lateral rotation or translation.
3 Correct the positional malalignment by applying either a medial or a lateral accessory rotating or translating glide to the phalanx and repeat the provocative movement.

4 A rotational taping technique may be used to reinforce the medial or lateral rotational force onto the phalanx.
5 Alternatively, a medial or lateral accessory glide force may be applied and reinforced with the tape.

6 Attach one end of the 19 mm strip of tape on the relevant phalanx, tension the tape and apply in the direction identified to benefit the patient's symptoms.
7 A lock-off tape may be applied over the dorsal or palmar aspect of the hand to lock the narrow strips in place.

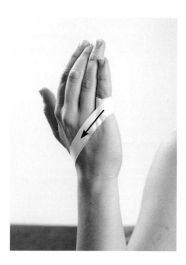

8 The provocative movement is repeated to ensure reduction in pain and/or increase in ROM is maintained.

9 Alternatively, elasticised tape may be used to perform the above techniques.

Reassessment

○ Circulation, patient comfort and symptoms at rest.

○ Passive and active restriction of ROM of finger flexion or extension.

○ Provocative movement of the finger and symptoms.

34

REFERENCES

Alexander, C M, Stynes, S, Thomas, A, Lewis, J and Harrison, P J (2003) Does tape facilitate or inhibit the lower fibres of trapezius? Manual Therapy, 8(1): 37–41.

Andrews, J R, Wilk, K E, et al (1993) Physical examination of the thrower's elbow. Journal of Orthopaedic & Sports Physical Therapy, 17(6): 296–304.

Bendre, A A, Hartigan, B J, et al (2005) Mallet finger. Journal of the American Academy of Orthopaedic Surgeons, 13(5): 336–44.

Brukner, P, Khan, K (2007) Clinical Sports Medicine. McGraw-Hill, Sydney.

Burkhart, S S, Lo, I K Y (2007) The CAM effect of the proximal humerus: its role in the production of relative capsular redundancy of the shoulder. Arthroscopy, 23(3): 241–6.

Cook, G S, Lalonde, D H (2008) MOC-PSSM CME article: management of thumb carpometacarpal joint arthritis. Plastic & Reconstructive Surgery, 121(1 Suppl): 1–9.

Coons, M S, Green, S M (1995) Boutonniere deformity. Hand Clinics, 11(3): 387–402.

Donatelli, R (2004) Physical Therapy of the Shoulder. Churchill Livingstone, St Louis, Missouri.

Edelstein, D M, Kardashian, G, et al (2008) Radial collateral ligament injuries of the thumb. Journal of Hand Surgery American Volume, 33(5): 760–70.

Falla, D, Bilenkij, G, Jull, G (2004) Patients with chronic neck pain demonstrate altered patterns of muscle activation during performance of a functional upper limb task. Spine, 29: 1436–40.

Folk, B (2001) Traumatic thumb injury management using mobilization with movement. Manual Therapy, 6(3): 178–82.

Greig, A M, Bennell, K L, et al (2008) Postural taping decreases thoracic kyphosis but does not influence trunk muscle electromyographic activity or balance in women with osteoporosis. Manual Therapy, 13(3): 249–57.

Guererro, P, Busconi, B, et al (2009) Congenital instability of the shoulder joint: assessment and treatment options. Journal of Orthopaedic & Sports Physical Therapy, 39(2): 124–34.

Hardy, M A (2004) Principles of metacarpal and phalangeal fracture management: a review of rehabilitation concepts. Journal of Orthopaedic & Sports Physical Therapy, 34(12): 781–99.

Hess, S (2000) Functional stability of the glenohumeral joint. Manual Therapy, 5(2): 63–7.

Ide, J, Kataoka, Y, et al (2003) Compression and stretching of the brachial plexus in thoracic outlet syndrome: correlation between neuroradiographic findings and symptoms and signs produced by provocation manoeuvres. J Hand Surg [Br], 28(3): 218–23.

Kibler, W B (2006) Scapular dysfunction. Athletic Therapy Today, 11(5): 6–9.

Kovacic, J, Bergfeld, J, et al (2005) Return to play issues in upper extremity injuries. Clinical Journal of Sport Medicine, 15(6): 448–52.

Lewis, J, Valentine, V (2007) The pectoralis minor length test: a study of the intra-rater reliability and diagnostic accuracy in subjects with and without shoulder symptoms. BMC Musculoskeletal Disorders, 8(64).

Lewis, J S, Wright, C, et al (2005) Subacromial impingement syndrome: the effect of changing posture on shoulder range of movement. Journal of Orthopaedic & Sports Physical Therapy, 35(2): 72–87.

Lorei, M P, Hershman, E B (1993) Peripheral-nerve injuries in athletes — treatment and prevention. Sports Medicine, 16(2): 130–47.

Marin, R (1998) Scapula winger's brace: a case series on the management of long thoracic nerve palsy. Archives of Physical Medicine & Rehabilitation, 79(10): 1226–30.

McConnell, J (2000) A novel approach to pain relief pre-therapeutic exercise. Journal of Science and Medicine in Sport, 3(3): 325–34.

McConnell, J, McIntosh, B (2009) The effect of tape on glenohumeral rotation range of motion in elite junior tennis players. Clinical Journal of Sport Medicine, 19(2): 90–4.

Morin, G, Tiberio, D, et al (1997) The effect of upper trapezius taping on electromyographic activity in the upper and middle trapezius region. Journal of Sport Rehabilitation, 6(4): 309–18.

Morrissey, D (2000) Proprioceptive shoulder taping. Journal of Bodywork and Movement Therapies, 4: 189–94.

Mulligan, B (1999) Manual therapy 'NAGS', 'SNAGS', 'MWMS' etc. Plane View Services, Wellington.

O'Leary, S, Carroll, M, et al (2002) The effect of soft tissue deloading tape on thoracic spine pressure pain thresholds in asymptomatic subjects. Manual Therapy, 7(3): 150–3.

Ofir, H N, Eyal, M (2007) Upper-extremity deep-vein thrombosis in an elderly man. Canadian Medical Association Journal, 176(8): 1078.

Pascarelli, E F, Hsu, Y P (2001) Understanding work-related upper extremity disorders: clinical findings in 485 computer users, musicians, and others. Journal of Occupational Rehabilitation, 11(1): 1–21.

Peterson, D, Blankenship, K, et al (1997) Investigation of the validity and reliability of four objective techniques for measuring forward shoulder posture. Journal of Orthopaedic & Sports Physical Therapy, 25(1): 34–41.

Peterson, J J, Bancroft, L W, et al (2006) Injuries of the fingers and thumb in the athlete. Clinics in Sports Medicine, 25(3): 527–42.

Poolman Rudolf, W, Goslings, J C, et al (2005) Conservative treatment for closed fifth (small finger) metacarpal neck fractures. Cochrane Database of Systematic Reviews. DOI: 10.1002/14651858.CD003210.pub3.

Prosser, R (1995) Conservative management of ulnar carpal instability. Australian Journal of Physiotherapy, 41(1): 41–6.

Sahrmann, S (2002) Diagnosis and Treatment of Movement Impairment Syndromes. Mosby, St Louis.

Selkowitz, D M, Chaney, C, Stuckey, S J, Vlad, G (2007) The effects of scapular taping on the surface electromyographic signal amplitude of shoulder girdle muscles during upper extremity elevation in individuals with suspected shoulder impingement syndrome. Journal of Orthopaedic & Sports Physical Therapy, 37(11): 694–702.

Shabat, S, Sagiv, P, et al (2002) Avulsion fracture of the flexor digitorum profundus tendon ('jersey finger') type III. Archives of Orthopaedic & Trauma Surgery, 122(3): 182–3.

Shamus, J L, Shamus, E C (1997) A taping technique for the treatment of acromioclavicular joint sprains: a case study. Journal of Orthopaedic & Sports Physical Therapy, 25(6): 390–4.

Shippert, B W (2007) A 'Complex jersey finger': case report and literature review. Clinical Journal of Sport Medicine, 17(4): 319–20.

Singletary, S, Freeland, A E, et al (2003) Metacarpal fractures in athletes: treatment, rehabilitation, and safe early return to play. Journal of Hand Therapy, 16(2): 171–9.

Staes, F F, Banks, K J, et al (2009) Reliability of accessory motion testing at the carpal joints. Manual Therapy, 14(3): 292–8.

Stoddard, J K, Johnson, C D (2000) Conservative treatment of a patient with a mild acromioclavicular joint separation. Journal of Sports Chiropractic & Rehabilitation, 14(4): 118–28.

Timm, K (1985) Pollex valgus: orthopaedic management for ulnar instability of the metacarpophalangeal joint of the thumb. Journal of Orthopaedic & Sports Physical Therapy, 6(6): 334–42.

Tuttle, H G, Olvey, S P, et al (2006) Tendon avulsion injuries of the distal phalanx. Clinical Orthopaedics & Related Research, 445: 157–68.

Vicenzino, B, Brooksbank, J, et al (2003) Initial effects of elbow taping on pain-free grip strength and pressure pain threshold. Journal of Orthopaedic & Sports Physical Therapy, 33(7): 400–7.

Vicenzino, B, Wright, A (1995) Effects of a novel manipulative physiotherapy technique on tennis elbow: a single case study. Manual Therapy, 1(1): 30–5.

Yamazaki, M, Kobayashi, N, et al (2005) Fixation in the extended position of the PIP joint with volar plate avulsion fracture: evaluation of ROM and bone union. Japanese Journal of Judo Therapy, 14(2): 81–8.

Young, D, Papp, S, et al (2007) Physical examination of the wrist. Orthopedic Clinics of North America, 38: 149–65.

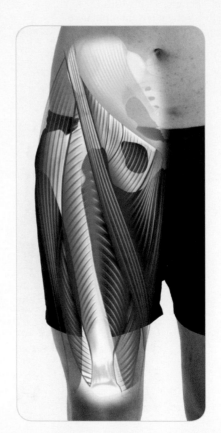
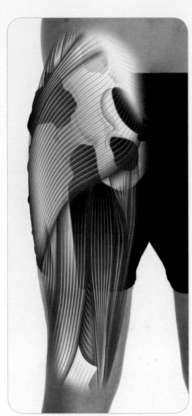
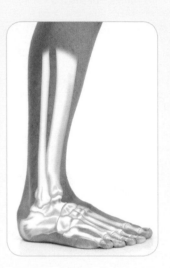
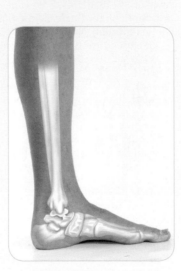

Hip joint and buttock

Greater trochanteric pain syndrome

Background and rationale

Greater trochanteric pain syndrome (GTPS) is an umbrella term that refers to a number of musculoskeletal conditions which include trochanteric bursitis and gluteus medius tendinitis or tendinopathy (Lievense et al 2005; Walker et al 2007). GTPS often presents with lateral hip pain symptoms and assessment findings may include iliotibial band (ITB) tenderness (Segal et al 2007), trochanteric bursa tenderness or gluteus medius pain. As an adjunct to usual conservative management, taping may be used to provide 'lateral support' to the hip, and decrease the load or stress placed on the trochanteric bursa or gluteus medius tendon by the iliotibial band at rest and during movement.

Evidence

- No research studies relating to this technique were identified.

Material

- Hypoallergenic underlay 2 × 20–40 cm strips.
- Rigid tape 14–16 × 20–40 cm strips.
- Blunt nose scissors.

Patient position

- Side-lying position with the uppermost leg being the affected side.
- Upper leg is placed in neutral hip position and in slight hip abduction, while resting on a pillow.

Therapist position

- Standing behind the patient.

35

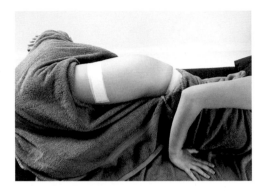

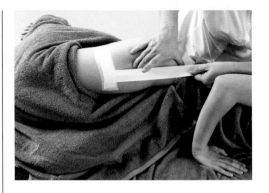

1 Apply one strip of hypoallergenic underlay from anterior superior iliac spine (ASIS) to posterior superior iliac spine (PSIS) in a horizontal direction.

2 Apply a second strip of hypoallergenic underlay horizontally across the top of the thigh, approximately 25 cm inferior to the greater trochanter.

3 Apply the first strip of tape over the inferior hypoallergenic underlay with one hand while gathering the tissues in a centred and upwards direction with the other hand. This strip of tape will act as the inferior anchor.

4 Apply the second strip of tape over the superior hypoallergenic underlay with one hand by gathering the tissues in a centred and downwards direction towards the greater trochanter with the other hand. This strip of tape will act as the superior anchor.

5 Apply a longitudinal strip of tape starting anteriorly from the inferior anchor. Tension and place the tape on the superior anchor with one hand, while gathering and deloading the tissues towards the greater trochanter with the other hand.

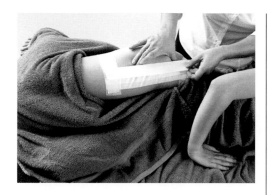

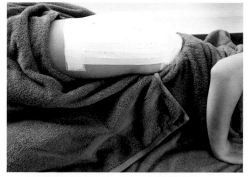

6 Repeat step 5 using approximately 8–12 strips of tape progressing from anterior to posterior direction overlapping each previous layer by half the width of the new layer.

7 Apply two strips of tape as lock-offs over the superior and inferior anchors, securing the longitudinal strips of tape in place.

Reassessment
○ Patient symptoms at rest.
○ Functional movements such as single leg stance, gait, sit to stand and symptoms experienced.

35

Limiting hip internal rotation

Background and rationale

Clinical assessment in patients with lower limb and pelvis conditions may reveal a positive Trendelenburg sign (Hardcastle & Nade 1985; Foucher et al 2007). This may be associated with increased hip internal rotation and/or adduction during single leg stance and gait as a result of weak or poorly activating hip external rotators and/or abductor muscles. As an adjunct to usual management, controlling the amount of abnormal femoral internal rotation and adduction during single leg stance or during gait may subsequently lead to lower limb symptom relief. This taping technique uses a single strip of tape placed in a spiral orientation around the hip to decrease abnormal hip internal rotation and adduction.

Evidence

○ No research studies relating to this technique were identified.

Material

○ Rigid tape 1 × 50 cm strip.

Patient position

○ Patient is lying in prone position with leg to be taped in figure-4 position.
○ Alternatively, patient may stand with one leg abducted and externally rotated at the hip, with the foot resting behind the knee.
○ Patient will need to be informed that it may be necessary for them to move their underwear slightly towards the sacrum to enable application of this technique.
○ Drape using a sheet or towel as necessary. Ensure adequate screening of the treatment area to allow for patient privacy.

Therapist position

○ Standing beside patient, on the side to be taped.

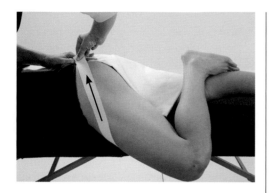

1 Start tape antero-medially at the mid thigh area.

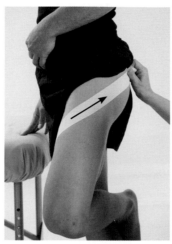

2 Direct the tape diagonally and slightly behind the hip joint to finish tape posteriorly to the buttock, near the sacrum.

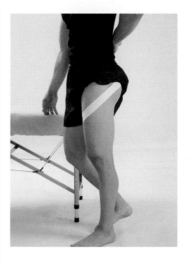

Reassessment
○ Symptoms in single leg stance and gait.
○ Effectiveness of tape to limit excessive hip internal rotation and adduction in stance phase.

36

Gluteus medius muscle facilitation

Background and rationale

Gluteus medius muscle weakness or altered motor activity may be implicated in lower limb conditions (Bewyer & Bewyer 2003) and may often be associated with a positive or reverse Trendelenburg sign during single leg stance and gait (Hardcastle & Nade 1985). Tape used as an adjunct to therapeutic exercise is proposed to facilitate the gluteus medius muscle activation during exercise.

Evidence

○ No research studies relating to this technique were identified.

Material

○ Rigid tape 5 × 15–20 cm strips and 2 × 5 cm strips (to be used as an anchor).
○ Hypoallergenic underlay 4 × 15–20 cm strips and 2 × 5 cm strips may be used (optional).

Patient position

○ Side-lying position, a pillow between the knees, hip approximately in 30° flexion and neutral abduction/adduction.
○ Patient should be informed that it may be necessary for them to move their underwear slightly towards the sacrum to enable application of this technique.
○ Drape using a sheet or towel as necessary. Ensure adequate screening of the treatment area to allow for patient privacy.

Therapist position

○ Standing beside the patient.

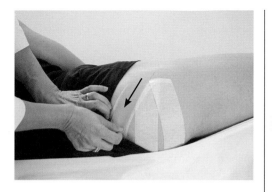 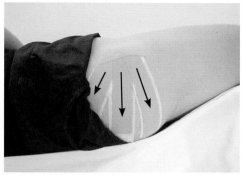

Reassessment

○ Symptoms in single leg stance and gait.
○ Therapeutic exercise for gluteus medius and patient-perceived ability to perform exercise.

1 Apply one strip of 5 cm hypoallergenic underlay over the greater trochanter to be used as the inferior anchor (optional).

2 Apply one strip of 5 cm tape over the greater trochanter to be used as the inferior anchor.

3 Apply one strip of 15 cm hypoallergenic underlay along the posterior inferior aspect of the iliac crest to act as the superior anchor (optional).

4 Apply one of the 15 cm strips of tape along the posterior inferior aspect of the iliac crest to act as the superior anchor (optional).

5 Apply a strip of 15 cm hypoallergenic underlay from the inferior anchor towards the superior anchor, without added pressure. The orientation of the hypoallergenic underlay should be in the same direction as the gluteus medius muscle fibres.

6 Repeat step 5 applying at least 3 strips of hypoallergenic underlay from the greater trochanter towards the iliac crest, over the direction of anterior, middle and posterior fibres of gluteus medius.

7 Apply one strip of 15 cm tape over the first hypoallergenic underlay, from the inferior anchor, tension and apply gently towards the superior anchor, without added pressure.

8 Repeat step 7, applying at least 3 strips of tape from the greater trochanter towards the iliac crest, over the hypoallergenic underlay in the direction of anterior, middle and posterior fibres of gluteus medius.

9 Apply a second 5 cm strip of tape over the greater trochanter to act as inferior tape lock-off.

10 Repeat step 2 using a second 15 cm strip of tape to act as the superior tape lock-off.

37

Gluteus medius muscle deloading

Background and rationale
Gluteus medius muscle tears or tendinopathy have been reported in the literature and are often associated with GTPS (Kingzett-Taylor et al 1999; Bewyer & Bewyer 2003). Taping aimed at unloading the painful gluteus medius muscle and tendon can be a useful adjunct to usual management of gluteus medius tears or tendinopathy. A variation to the previous technique is used, incorporating the tissue deloading principles for taping.

Evidence
- No research studies relating to this technique were identified.

Material
- Rigid tape 8×15–20 cm strips and 2×5 cm strips (to be used as anchors).
- Hypoallergenic underlay 6×15–20 cm strips and 2×5 cm strips may be used (optional).

Patient position
- Side-lying position, a pillow between the knees, hip approximately in 30° flexion and neutral abduction/adduction.
- Patient should be informed that it may be necessary for them to move their underwear slightly towards the sacrum to enable application of this technique.
- Drape using a sheet or towel as necessary. Ensure adequate screening of the treatment area to allow for patient privacy.

Therapist position
- Standing beside the patient.

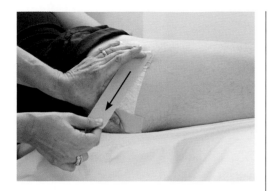

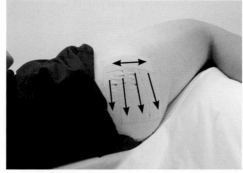

1 Apply one strip of 5 cm tape over the greater trochanter to be used as the inferior anchor.
2 Apply one of the 15 cm strips of tape along the posterior aspect of the iliac crest to act as the superior anchor.
3 Apply a strip of 15 cm tape from the inferior anchor, tensioning with one hand while gathering the tissues inwards and towards the centre of the iliac fossa with the other hand.
4 Place tape on the superior anchor. The orientation of the tape should be in the same direction as the gluteus medius muscle fibres.

5 Repeat step 3, with a further 4–5 strips of 15 cm tape, overlapping the previous layer of tape by half the width of each new layer of tape, while deloading the tissues each time.
6 Apply a second 5 cm strip of tape over the greater trochanter to act as inferior tape lock-off.
7 Repeat step 2 using a second 15 cm strip of tape to act as the superior tape lock-off.
8 Hypoallergenic underlay may be applied under the technique prior to application of tape (optional).

Reassessment
○ Symptoms in single leg stance and gait.
○ Provocative movement (Kingzett-Taylor et al 1999).

38

Gluteus maximus muscle facilitation

Background and rationale
Changes in gluteus maximus muscle function have been reported in patients with low back pain (Leinonen et al 2000) and lower limb musculoskeletal conditions (Bullock-Saxton 1994; Grimaldi et al 2009). Management of patients with altered gluteus maximus function may include therapeutic exercises aimed at increasing the muscle activation. Taping may be used as an adjunct to therapeutic exercise, aiming to activate gluteus maximus in the early stages and to provide increased patient awareness of the muscle activation with a proposed facilitatory effect.

Evidence
○ No research studies relating to this technique were identified.

Material
○ Rigid tape 10 × 15–20 cm strips.
○ Hypoallergenic underlay 10 × 15–20 cm strips may be used (optional).

Patient position
○ Prone.
○ Alternative position: standing with pelvis in neutral position.

Therapist position
○ Standing beside the patient on the side of the leg to be taped if patient is lying down, or standing behind the patient if the patient is standing up.

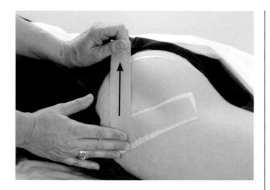

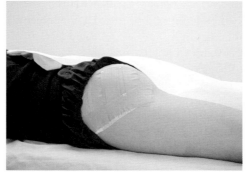

1 Apply the first strip of tape close to the gluteus maximus insertion on the lateral border of the iliotibial band (ITB), from distal to proximal to act as the distal anchor.

2 Apply a second strip of tape on the medial border of the buttock, from distal to proximal, to act as the proximal anchor.

3 Apply a strip of tape from the distal to the proximal anchor and laterally to medially, laying tape gently along the fibre direction of the gluteus maximus.

4 Repeat with several strips of tape, gently laying them along the fibres of the gluteus maximus, allowing a small gap between the layers of tape.

5 Repeat steps 1 and 2, using two strips of tape to lock-off the gluteal tape over the superior and inferior anchors.

6 Hypoallergenic underlay may be applied and laid gently on the skin under the technique prior to application of tape (optional).

Reassessment
○ Patient comfort and any symptoms at rest.
○ Therapeutic exercise requiring gluteus maximus activation.

39

Buttock and sciatica pain deloading

Background and rationale

The following taping technique was first described by Jenny McConnell as a novel approach to providing pain relief in patients experiencing sciatic pain (McConnell 2000; McConnell 2002) proposing to unload the structures of the S1 region. Clinically this technique has been found to be effective in reducing symptoms of sciatica. The proposed effects of the taping technique are to unload the muscles overlying the neural tissues such as the glutei (and piriformis), hamstrings and gastroc/soleus muscle groups, however, the definitive effects are still uncertain and will remain speculative until conclusive research is conducted.

In a study by Kilbreath et al (2006) the same gluteal taping technique was used in a randomised cross-over design study in 15 participants who previously had a stroke. The authors found that hip extension ROM increased significantly during gait when the gluteal taping was applied. The authors noted that the trunk was more upright in patients when taped, facilitating the maintenance of a neutral rather than flexed position of the pelvis which in turn assisted the hip extensors to produce a greater extension moment.

Evidence

○ No research studies relating to this technique for the treatment of sciatica were identified.
○ Kilbreath et al (2006) determined that this technique increased hip extension in stroke patients (Level IV).

Material

○ Hypoallergenic underlay 5 × 20 cm strips.
○ Rigid tape 5 × 20 cm strips.

Patient position

○ Prone.
○ Alternative position: standing (with support to hold onto if needed) with pelvis in neutral position.

Therapist position

○ Standing beside the patient on the side of the leg to be taped if patient is lying down, or standing behind if the patient is standing up.

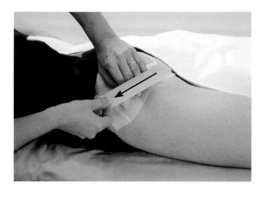 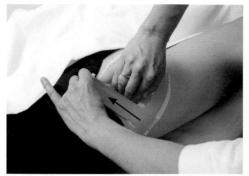 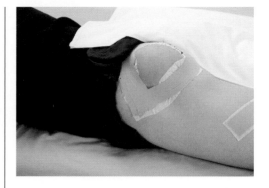

1 Apply the first strip of hypoallergenic underlay along the inferior gluteal fold from medial to lateral.
2 Apply a second strip of hypoallergenic underlay along the superior border of gluteus maximus, along the line of the iliac crest.
3 Apply the third strip of hypoallergenic underlay along the medial gluteal line from inferior to superior so that the hypoallergenic underlay strips join together and form a triangle.
4 Apply the first strip of rigid tape along the inferior gluteal fold on the medial side and while tensioning the tape with one hand gather the soft tissues towards the centre of the buttock with the other hand and apply the tensioned tape on the lateral side of the gluteal fold, following the hypoallergenic underlay.
5 Apply a second strip of tape along the iliac crest on the superior border of gluteus maximus over the hypoallergenic underlay while, similar to step 4, the soft tissues are gathered and lifted towards the centre of the buttock.

6 Apply a third strip of tape along the medial gluteal line over the hypoallergenic underlay while similarly gathering and lifting the soft tissues towards the middle of the buttock.
7 The tape should look like a triangle around the contours of gluteus maximus and the skin should have a puckered appearance.

40

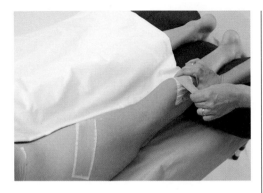
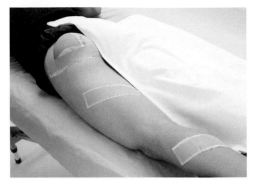

8 If the sciatica pain radiates down the posterior aspect of the thigh and/or the calf, an oblique strip of tape may be applied over the hamstrings and the calf muscles. The tape is applied with one hand while the other hand is gathering the tissues together towards the middle of the tape. Hypoallergenic underlay may be applied underneath this additional strip of tape if preferred.

Reassessment
○ Comfort of tape and symptoms at rest.
○ Lumbar spine ROM if symptomatic.
○ Neural tissue provocation test for sciatic nerve such as straight leg raise if indicated.

40

Adductor muscle deloading

Background and rationale

Adductor muscle strains or tears near the groin area (Strauss et al 2007) and adductor tendon insertion injuries are common, particularly in athletes (Nicholas & Tyler 2002), and may be associated with pain and limited function (Biedert et al 2003). Tape may be used to unload the adductor muscles close to their insertion with the proposed effect of reducing strain on the injured or painful structures and thus decreasing the symptoms of pain.

Evidence

- No research studies relating to this technique were identified.

Material

- Rigid tape 1 × 30 cm strip.

Patient position

- Patient is standing with the feet evenly apart. A heel lift of approximately 4 cm is used on the side to be treated.
- Patient is wearing shorts or underwear to allow access for the taping.

Therapist position

- Sitting in front of the patient.

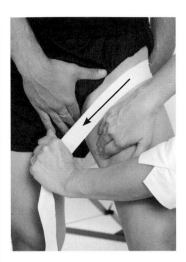

1 Start the tape on the lateral aspect of the thigh, near the greater trochanter. Tension the tape with one hand as it is being placed over the anterior thigh.
2 Direct the tape towards the medial aspect of the thigh and while holding the tension of the tape with one hand, gather the tissues over the adductor muscles inwards and upwards towards the adductor muscle insertion with the other hand. Place the tape under the gathered tissues.

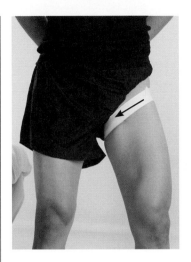

3 Continue with the tape over the posterior thigh and finish tape on the lateral aspect of the thigh.

Reassessment

- Adductor muscle test contraction or stretching.
- Walking and other provocative activity.

Thigh

Box taping technique for cork thigh, muscle haematomas and muscle strains/tears

Background and rationale

Traumatic injuries to the muscles may result in contusions, tears or strains and be associated with pain and inflammation (Matzkin et al 2007), limited muscle activation and extensibility and increased functional limitation. Initial management of acute injuries will depend on the patient, the severity of the injury, the inflammatory response and the phase of healing and repair (Matzkin et al 2007) and will vary depending on the muscle group.

As an adjunct to the usual management of muscle injuries, deloading tape may be used to unload the injured structures. Using tape to unload injured or painful soft tissues has been documented in a number of techniques in this book, with the purported effects outlined in Chapter 2. As outlined, a number of clinical case reports have described the use of unloading taping techniques, though research in the area is scarce (O'Leary et al 2002).

The box taping technique may be used therapeutically as part of the management of muscle and soft tissues injuries in many regions of the body. It is not intended to be used for return-to-sport management after an acute injury. The technique described in this section is using a quadriceps haematoma as an example.

Evidence

○ No research studies relating to this technique were identified.
○ Box taping techniques have been described that have effectively reduced pain in other areas, for example the thoracic spine (O'Leary et al 2002), and in cases of elbow lateral epicondylalgia (Vicenzino et al 2003). The outcomes of these studies are described in more detail in Chapter 2.

Material

○ Hypoallergenic underlay may be used if preferred.
○ Rigid tape 8 × 15–20 cm strips.

Patient position

○ Supine, with knee resting on a rolled towel at about 20–30° flexion.
○ For this procedure, if the area to be taped is hairy it would be preferable to shave or clip the hair, as the tape will adhere and be much more effective on a hairless area.

Therapist position

○ Standing beside the patient.

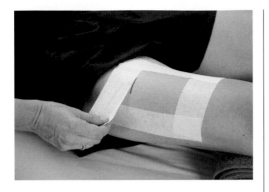

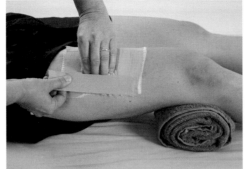

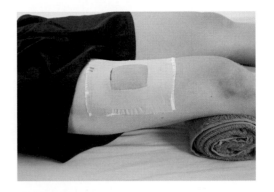

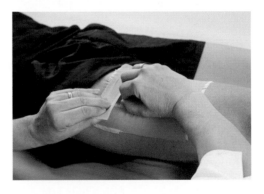

1 Identify the region of tenderness on the muscle by palpating inferior to the painful area and progressing towards the painful area. Use a pen to mark a line where tenderness of the soft tissues is first noted.

2 Repeat step 1 for the lateral, medial and superior sides of the injured area to form a 'square' or a 'box' around the painful or injured tissues.

3 If hypoallergenic underlay is to be used apply it in a square, over the markings drawn around the injured tissues or haematoma.

4 Apply a strip of tape on the inferior side of the square, tension it with one hand and while the other hand is gathering and drawing the tissues towards the centre of the 'square', place it on the skin.

5 Apply the other three strips around the square in a similar manner, while ensuring the injured tissues are gently gathered towards the centre of the square. The tissues in the centre of the square should have a puckered effect.

6 Apply a second layer of tape in a similar manner, overlapping the previous layer by half the width of the new layer of tape. With the new layer of tape the tissues in the centre of the square should have an increased puckered look.

Reassessment

For quadriceps contusion:

○ symptoms at rest

○ pain-free active ROM: knee flexion and extension

○ walking, provocative activity and symptoms.

42

Vastus lateralis muscle inhibitory taping (and iliotibial band deloading)

Background and rationale

In patients with patellofemoral pain syndrome (PFPS) the vastus lateralis (VL) and vastus medialis obliquus (VMO) muscle activation and timing difference during functional tasks has been well documented (Cowan et al 2002). If the treatment aim in PFPS is to inhibit increased activity of VL muscle this may be achieved using a taping technique that incorporates tape applied firmly across the muscle fibres of the muscle. This technique, first described by Jenny McConnell in a course handbook (cited by Tobin & Robinson 2000), has been shown to be effective in VL inhibition in asymptomatic subjects during a functional task (McCarthy Persson et al 2008). It is important to be reminded that VL muscle anatomically lies under the iliotibial band (ITB) and these structures are thus intricately related. Assessment of the ITB is usually included in lower limb conditions and it may be found to be taut or tight. In particular, using the Ober test to assess the ITB, it has been shown to be tighter in PFPS patients (Hudson & Darthuy 2006; Hudson 2009). The following taping technique is used as an adjunct to usual treatment and proposes to decrease VL activity in patients with knee conditions where this is indicated, and it may also have a subsequent effect on symptoms related to ITB tightness. The effect of this taping technique on lower limb symptoms related to ITB tightness has not been investigated. Immediate effect of the taping on symptoms will give the therapist a good indication as to the success of the technique.

Evidence

○ This technique has been shown to decrease VL muscle activity in asymptomatic participants (Tobin & Robinson 2000; McCarthy Persson et al 2008) (Level IV).

Material

○ Hypoallergenic underlay 3 × 15 cm strips.
○ Rigid tape 3 × 15 cm strips.

Patient position

○ Supine with knee resting on a rolled towel in slight knee flexion.

Therapist position

○ Standing beside the patient on the side to be taped.

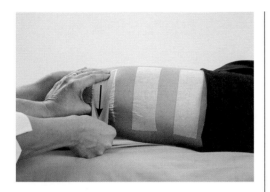

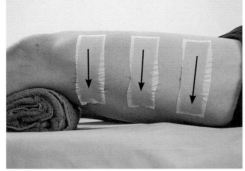

1 Apply 3 strips of hypoallergenic underlay across the VL muscle fibres starting approximately 5 cm superior to the knee joint line, and then 5–10 cm apart from distal to proximal.

2 Apply a strip of tape over the first hypoallergenic underlay on the anterior aspect of the thigh, and while tensioning the tape with one hand gather the VL tissues towards the middle of the hypoallergenic underlay with the other hand and place tape from medial to lateral direction. This applies a firm pressure over the VL and ITB.

3 Repeat step 2 with a second strip of tape laying it over the middle strip of hypoallergenic underlay.

4 Repeat step 2 with a third strip of tape laying it over the most proximal strip of hypoallergenic tape.

Reassessment

○ Comfort and symptoms including patellofemoral pain at rest.

○ VMO muscle activation during knee extension or during a functional task.

○ Other lower limb symptoms associated with VL increased activity or ITB tightness.

43

Knee joint

Iliotibial band (ITB) friction syndrome deloading

Background and rationale

Iliotibial band friction syndrome (ITBFS), commonly seen in runners and cyclists, is thought to be caused by increased strain and friction of the ITB over the lateral femoral epicondyle during knee flexion/extension movement (Ross et al 2007) at about 30° knee flexion (Brukner & Khan 2007). It has been argued that the symptoms of ITBFS may be more associated with pressure and compression of a layer of fat that lies underneath the ITB tract rather than friction of the band itself during flexion and extension of the knee (Fairclough et al 2006). Whatever the exact cause of the localised symptoms over the lateral femoral epicondyle is, using tape to unload the structures as an adjunct to usual treatment may provide the patient with temporary symptomatic relief.

Evidence

○ No research studies relating to this technique were identified.

Material

○ Hypoallergenic underlay 2 × 5–10 cm strips.
○ Rigid tape 2 × 5–10 cm strips.

Patient position

○ Supine with knee resting on a rolled towel in 30° knee flexion.

Therapist position

○ Standing beside the patient on the side to be taped.

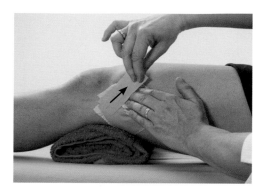

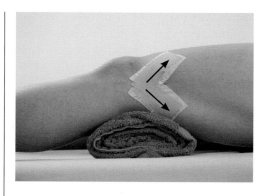

1 Identify the lateral femoral epicondyle and the tender area where the patient is experiencing their symptoms.

2 Apply a strip of hypoallergenic underlay inferior to the lateral femoral epicondyle, from medial to lateral.

3 Apply a second strip of hypoallergenic underlay inferior to the lateral femoral epicondyle, from lateral to medial, forming a 'V' shape around the lateral femoral epicondyle.

4 Apply a strip of tape inferior to the lateral femoral epicondyle immediately over the hypoallergenic underlay. Tension the tape with one hand and, while lifting and gathering the soft tissues towards the centre of the 'V' with the other hand, apply the tape from medial to lateral.

5 Apply a second strip of tape inferior to the lateral femoral epicondyle, from lateral to medial, repeating step 4, lifting the gathered tissues towards the centre of the 'V'. Care should be taken with this strip not to place the tape too close to the patella as it may cause discomfort during its movement.

6 The finished tape should look like a 'V' around the lateral femoral epicondyle.

Reassessment

○ Comfort and symptoms at rest.

○ Provocative active knee movement, functional tasks and symptoms.

Pes anserinus bursitis/tendinopathy deloading

Background and rationale

Pes anserinus is the common tendinous insertion on the tibia of three muscles: gracilis, sartorius and semitendinosus. The pes anserinus bursa lies between the tibia and the common tendinous insertion (Brukner & Khan 2007) and may become inflamed from increased compression or friction of the overlying common tendon, leading to symptoms of bursitis. Pes anserinus tendinopathy could present with localised tenderness over the insertion point of pes anserinus. For each of these conditions tape may be used to unload the insertion of the pes anserine tendon.

Evidence

○ No research studies relating to this technique were identified.

Material

○ Hypoallergenic underlay 2 × 5–10 cm strips.
○ Rigid tape 2 × 5–10 cm strips.

Patient position

○ Supine with knee resting on a rolled towel in slight knee flexion.

Therapist position

○ Standing beside the patient on the side to be taped.

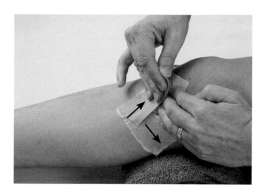

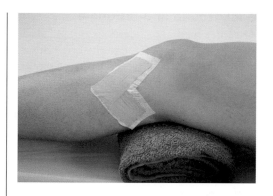

1 Identify the common insertional tendon of pes anserinus and the tender area on the medial aspect of the tibia where the patient is experiencing their symptoms.

2 Apply a strip of hypoallergenic underlay inferior to the insertion of pes anserinus, from medial to lateral.

3 Apply a second strip of hypoallergenic underlay inferior to the insertion of pes anserinus, from lateral to medial, forming a 'V' shape around the insertion of pes anserinus.

4 Apply a strip of tape inferior to the insertion of pes anserinus immediately over the hypoallergenic underlay. Tension the tape with one hand and while lifting and gathering the soft tissues towards the centre of the 'V' with the other hand, apply the tape from medial to lateral.

5 Apply a second strip of tape inferior to the insertion of pes anserinus, from lateral to medial, lifting the gathered tissues towards the centre of the 'V'. Care should be taken with this strip not to place the tape too close to the patella as it may cause discomfort during its movement.

6 The finished tape should look like a 'V' around the insertion of pes anserinus.

Reassessment
○ Comfort and symptoms at rest.
○ Provocative active knee movement, functional tasks and symptoms.

Knee medial collateral ligament (MCL) or medial meniscus injury

Background and rationale

The knee medial collateral ligament (MCL) sprain is usually caused by a valgus force to the knee either in contact or non-contact sports or activities. The severity of the injury is classified in grades I–III and the symptoms of pain, inflammation and functional limitation will vary based on the grade of the injury (Brukner & Khan 2007). Tape may be used as an adjunct to usual management of the injured ligament at any stage of the healing cycle to provide support to the medial knee. The aim of the treatment is to reduce the mechanical stress on the healing ligament. For this reason tape is applied in such a way as to replicate the function of the ligament it is designed to support.

The same taping technique described below may also prove beneficial in cases of medial meniscus injury, as it does provide pressure and support over the medial joint line.

Evidence

○ No research studies relating to this technique were identified.

Material

○ Hypoallergenic underlay 2 × 40–60 cm strips, optional.
○ Rigid tape 4 × 40–60 cm strips (depending on the size of the patient's quadriceps and calf muscle circumference).
○ Rigid tape 6 × 20–30 cm strips (depending on the size of the patient).

Patient position

○ Standing with heel resting on a 5 cm roll (usually a tape roll may suffice) and knee in approximately 30° flexion.

Therapist position

○ Sitting on a stool or chair, in front of the patient.

1 To apply the superior anchor, first ask the patient to statically contract their quadriceps muscle, and apply the tape over the contracted quadriceps, generally 10–15 cm above the knee joint line. This will ensure the circumferential anchor will accommodate the contracted muscle and will not cause discomfort during movement. Ensure the ends of the tape are superimposed in an oblique direction to avoid a tourniquet effect.

2 To apply the inferior anchor, ask the patient to statically contract their gastrocnemius/soleus muscles, and apply the tape over the contracted muscles, generally 10–15 cm below the knee joint line.

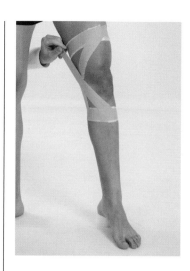
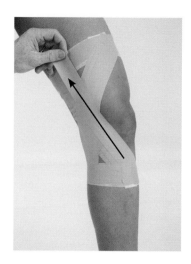

Apply the six strips of tape medially over the ligament as follows:

3 Apply the first strip starting on the inferior anchor posteriorly and direct it obliquely and superiorly so that it crosses the joint line slightly posterior to the anatomical position of MCL and finishes anteriorly on the superior anchor.

4 Apply the second strip of tape starting on the inferior anchor anteriorly and direct it obliquely and superiorly so that it crosses the joint line slightly posterior to the MCL and finishes on the superior anchor posteriorly. The two strips of tape should form an 'X' over the medial knee joint line.

5 Repeat steps 3 and 4 with a second pair of tape strips. Start each strip of tape on the inferior anchor overlapping the previous strip of tape with half the width, crossing the joint line over the anatomical position of MCL. The two strips of tape should form the 'X' over the medial knee joint line and over the MCL.

46

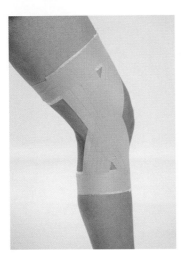

6 Repeat steps 3 and 4 with a third pair of tape strips. Start on the inferior anchor overlapping the previous strips of tape by half a width and crossing the joint line anterior to the MCL. The two strips of tape should form the 'X' over the medial knee joint line, slightly anterior to the MCL. Care must be taken with the last pair of tape strips to ensure they are not in contact with the patella, possibly interfering with its function.

7 Apply two lock-off anchors over the superior and inferior anchors in the same way as in steps 1 and 2 above.

8 For injuries where oedema is an issue, an elasticised support bandage worn over the taping technique may also be indicated.

Reassessment
- Comfort and symptoms at rest.
- Symptoms during gait, including patient's confidence with movement.
- Sporting drills or skills (if the taping technique is performed in the rehabilitation phase when the athlete is returning back to sport).

Knee lateral collateral ligament (LCL) or lateral meniscus injury

Background and rationale

The knee lateral collateral ligament (LCL) sprain is less common than the medial collateral ligament (MCL) and is usually caused by a large direct varus force to the knee either in contact or non-contact sports or activities. The severity of the injury is classified in grades I–III and the symptoms of pain, inflammation and functional limitation will vary based on the grade of the injury (Brukner & Khan 2007). Tape may be used as an adjunct to usual management of the injured ligament at any stage of the healing cycle to provide support to the lateral knee. The aim of the treatment is to reduce the mechanical stress on the healing ligament. For this reason tape is applied in such a way as to replicate the function of the ligament it is designed to support.

The same taping technique described below may also prove beneficial in cases of lateral meniscus injury, as it does provide pressure and support over the lateral joint line.

Evidence

○ No research studies relating to this technique were identified.

Material

○ Hypoallergenic underlay 2 × 40–60 cm strips, optional.
○ Rigid tape 4 × 40–60 cm strips (depending on the size of the patient's quadriceps and calf muscle circumference).
○ Rigid tape 6 × 20–30 cm strips (depending on the height of the patient).

Patient position

○ Standing with heel resting on a 5 cm roll and knee in approximately 30° flexion.

Therapist position

○ Sitting on a stool or chair, in front of the patient.

1 To apply the superior anchor, first ask the patient to statically contract their quadriceps muscle, and apply the tape over the contracted quadriceps, generally 10–15 cm above the knee joint line. This will ensure the circumferential anchor will accommodate the contracted muscle and will not cause discomfort during movement. Ensure the ends of the tape are superimposed in an oblique direction to avoid the tourniquet effect.

2 To apply the inferior anchor, ask the patient to statically contract their gastrocnemius/soleus muscles, and apply the tape over the contracted muscles, generally 10–15 cm below the knee joint line.

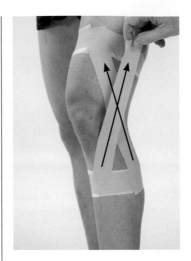

Apply the six strips of tape laterally over the ligament as follows:

3 Apply the first strip starting on the inferior anchor posteriorly and direct it obliquely and superiorly so that it crosses the joint line slightly posterior to the anatomical position of LCL and finishes anteriorly on the superior anchor.

4 Apply the second strip of tape starting on the inferior anchor anteriorly and direct it obliquely and superiorly so that it crosses the joint line slightly posterior to the LCL and finishes on the superior anchor posteriorly. The two strips of tape should form an 'X' over the lateral knee joint line.

5 Repeat steps 3 and 4 with a second pair of tape strips, starting each strip of tape on the inferior anchor overlapping half a width of the previous strip of tape, this time crossing the joint line over the anatomical position of the LCL. The two strips of tape should form the 'X' over the lateral knee joint line and over the LCL.

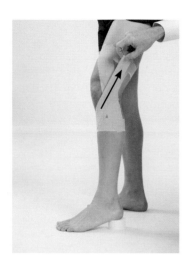

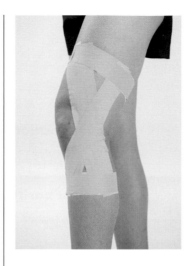

6 Repeat steps 3 and 4 with a third pair of tape strips, starting on the inferior anchor overlapping half a width of the previous strips of tape, this time crossing the joint line anterior to the LCL. The two strips of tape should form the 'X' over the lateral knee joint line, slightly anterior to the LCL. Care must be taken with the last pair of tape strips to ensure they are not in contact with the patella, possibly interfering with its function.

7 Apply two lock-off anchors over the superior and inferior anchors in the same ways as in steps 1 and 2 above.

8 For injuries where oedema is an issue, an elasticised support bandage worn over the taping technique may also be indicated.

Reassessment

○ Comfort and symptoms at rest.
○ Symptoms during gait, including patient's confidence with movement.
○ Sporting drills or skills (if the taping technique is performed in the rehabilitation phase when the athlete is returning back to sport).

47

Taping for anterior cruciate ligament (ACL) injury or to prevent knee hyperextension

Background and rationale

Anterior cruciate ligament (ACL) injuries are common in both contact and non-contact sports, and they are usually as a result of a pivoting/twisting action, when landing from a jump or during sudden deceleration. They may occur in conjunction with other injuries such as medial collateral ligament (MCL) sprain or a meniscus tear (Brukner & Khan 2007). The function of the ACL is inherent to the passive stability of the knee and prevents the tibia from translating anteriorly on the femur and controls rotational motion at the knee. The following taping technique aims to prevent the anterior translation of the tibia on the femur, possibly decreasing further strain on the injured ligament. It may be used as an adjunct to usual management of grade I or grade II ACL sprains to prevent further stress and damage, or in grade III injuries to minimise added motion of the tibia that may lead to meniscal irritation.

This taping technique has the added advantage of preventing hyperextension of the knee, which makes it a useful technique when control of knee hyperextension is a treatment aim.

Evidence

○ No research studies relating to this technique were identified.

Material

○ Rigid tape 1 × 80–100 cm strip (depending on the size of the patient's quadriceps muscle circumference and height).
○ Small square of 4 × 4 cm soft high-density foam (to be used as padding in the popliteal fossa — optional).

Patient position

○ Standing with leg to be taped in slight lunge position with approximately 20° knee flexion.

Therapist position

○ Squatting or sitting on a stool or chair, in front of the patient.

48

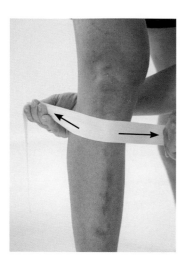

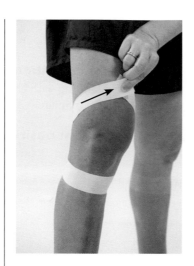

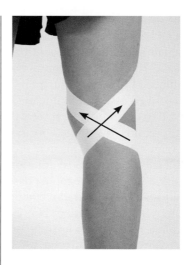

1 Place the centre of the long strip of tape over the tibial tuberosity.

2 Tensioning the tape on either side of the tibial tuberosity, direct and place it posterior to the knee, crossing the two sides of the tape over the posterior joint line over the optional pad, which can be added posteriorly to protect the structures behind the knee from the tape pressure.

3 Bring the two ends of the tape from posterior to anterior onto the thigh and, as the patient is gently extending the knee to full extension, lock off the two ends of tape on the anterior aspect of the thigh, slightly obliquely over each other.

4 The overall application of this taping technique is as a figure-of-8.

5 For injuries where oedema is an issue, an elasticised support bandage worn over the taping technique may be indicated.

Reassessment

○ Comfort and symptoms at rest.
○ Symptoms during gait, including patient's confidence with movement.
○ Sporting drills or skills (if the taping technique is performed in the rehabilitation phase when the athlete is returning back to sport).

Background and rationale

During knee assessment therapists may find that in certain conditions reducing the amount of internal or external tibial rotation decreases the patient's symptoms of pain and/or limited ROM. A technique of tibial rotation mobilisation with movement (MWM) as described by Brian Mulligan (1999) may be used to ascertain reduction of symptoms. If the MWM is effective, tape can be used to reinforce the rotated position of the tibia that provided the symptom relief. This may prove to be beneficial in managing residual symptoms post anterior cruciate ligament (ACL) or meniscal injuries. The taping described in this section is a spiral technique and it is used to facilitate tibial external rotation and limit internal rotation. However, applied in the reverse direction it will serve to facilitate tibial internal rotation and limit external rotation (Mulligan 1999).

Evidence

○ No research studies relating to this technique were identified.

Material

○ Rigid tape 1 × 60–80 cm strip (depending on patient's height).

Patient position

○ Standing with leg to be taped in slight lunge position with approximately 20° knee flexion.

Therapist position

○ Squatting or sitting on a stool or chair, in front of the patient.

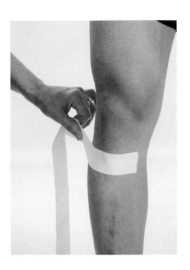

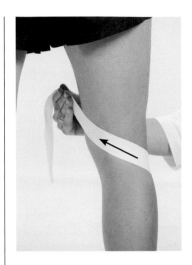

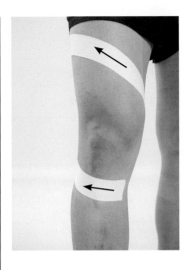

1 Apply one end of the tape approximately 2 cm medial to the tibial tuberosity.

2 Apply a rotation glide on the tibia with one hand and tensioning the tape apply it obliquely from medial to lateral direction, with the tape crossing the knee joint.

3 Bring the tape from posterior to the knee, finishing above the knee on the medial thigh.

49

Reassessment
- Comfort and symptoms at rest.
- Provocative movement, such as gait and symptoms.

Patellofemoral joint (PFJ)

PFJ position

Background and rationale

Patellofemoral pain syndrome (PFPS) or chondromalacia patella is a common condition (Callaghan & Selfe 2007) generally associated with antero-medial or infrapatellar pain and functional limitation (Brukner & Khan 2007), particularly on stairs and while squatting. The treatment approaches for PFPS have been described extensively in the literature, with the majority of studies investigating the use of tape as an adjunct to usual management, which includes exercise and manual therapy (Crossley et al 2002; Bennell et al 2005). A brief literature review on the use of tape in PFPS and its associated proposed effects is discussed in more detail in Chapter 2.

The following taping technique was first described by Jenny McConnell in 1986 and it requires the therapist to initially assess the position of the patella (Brukner & Khan 2007) and ascertain if medially gliding the patella, rotating, or tilting it provides symptom relief. This technique as described by McConnell (1986) has been investigated in various studies, some of which included the medial glide of the patella alone or in combination with tilting. It has also been investigated in patellofemoral osteoarthritis (OA) patients and found to be effective in reducing pain and in effecting a change in the patella position (Crossley et al 2009).

Evidence

○ The use of patella taping may: (i) reduce pain in the short term although the mechanism is unknown; (ii) be beneficial in conjunction with physiotherapy; (iii) alter VMO activity; and (iv) increase quadriceps strength. However, patella taping does not appear to alter patella congruence (Overington et al 2006) (Level I).
○ Patella taping reduces pain and disability in patients with knee OA (Hinman et al 2003) (Level II).
○ Tape in conjunction with exercise was effective in reducing pain in patellofemoral pain subjects (McConnell 1986) (Level IV).
○ The effectiveness of patella taping on vastus medialis obliquus (VMO) muscle facilitation or vastus lateralis (VL) inhibition is inconclusive (Bennell et al 2006; Cowan et al 2006; Keet et al 2007; Fagan & Delahunt 2008) (Levels IV, III-2, III-1, I).
○ Tape applied to VMO with stretch may increase VMO motor unit firing rate (Macgregor et al 2005) (Level IV).

Material

○ Hypoallergenic underlay 1 × 15–20 cm strip.
○ Rigid tape 3 × 10–12 cm strips.

Patient position

○ Supine with knee resting on a rolled towel in approximately 20–30° knee flexion.

Therapist position

○ Standing beside the patient.

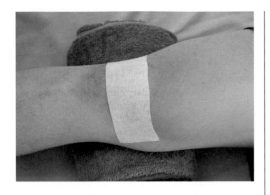 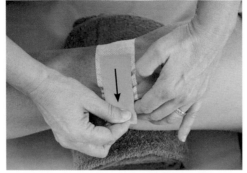 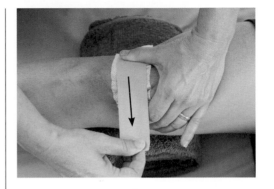

1 Apply hypoallergenic underlay tape horizontally over the patella, ensuring it reaches approximately 5 cm past the medial and lateral borders of the patella.

2 If patella is laterally tilted, the aim is to correct the lateral tilt first; apply a strip of tape on the centre of the patella and tension the tape to tilt the patella medially with one hand while gathering the medial tissues of the knee upwards with the other hand and apply tape on the medial aspect of the knee.

3 Correct with medial patellar glide next; apply a strip of tape laterally over the hypoallergenic underlay, tension the tape with one hand and while gliding the patella medially with the thumb of the other hand, gather the medial tissues upwards and apply the tape on the medial aspect of the knee.

50

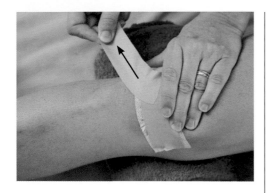

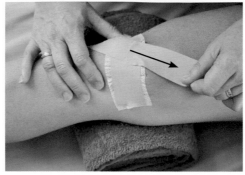

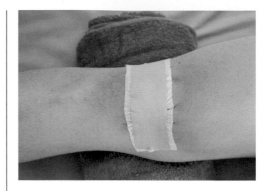

4 If the inferior pole of the patella is rotated medially or laterally, the aim is to correct the patellar rotation next; apply a piece of tape at the inferior pole of the patella, tension the tape and apply a rotational force laterally if the inferior pole is medial to the tibial tuberosity and medially if it rests lateral to the tibial tuberosity to correct the alignment. If further reinforcement of the rotation is required a strip of tape counter-rotating the patella is applied on the superior border of the patella.

5 When the technique is completed (with or without the rotational tape) support the tape on each side of the knee using the therapist's hands and ask the patient to actively flex the knee, while ensuring the tape adheres laterally and medially during the movement. This will enhance the tape adhesion.

6 Steps 2, 3 and 4 may also be performed in isolation from each other or in a combination of steps 2 and 3 or steps 3 and 4, depending on the findings of the patella position assessment and the relief of the patient's symptoms.

Reassessment
○ Comfort and symptoms at rest.
○ Patient's provocative movement such as gait or stepping down from a step and symptoms after each patellar correction component is ideal.

Patella fat pad deloading

Background and rationale

The patella fat pad is a highly vascularised structure that may be a source of patellofemoral pain that may become inflamed, tender and swollen if it is impinged under the inferior pole of the patella (Brukner & Khan 2007). The patella fat pad may usually be symptomatic on knee extension, or cause pain on heel strike during gait, or become symptomatic after knee arthroscopy (due to the entry point of the arthroscope).

This taping technique was first used by Jenny McConnell and reported in a case report in 2000 (McConnell 2000). Since then it has been adapted by many clinicians and described in part in several texts (Brukner & Khan 2007). The technique utilises the deloading principles to unload the painful fat pad by tilting the patella anteriorly and reducing the inferior pole impingement on the fat pad.

Evidence

- Patellar taping which may include a variation of the use of taping to unload the patella fat pad was found beneficial in reducing pain and disability in participants with knee OA (Hinman et al 2003) (Level II).
- A study by Crossley et al (2009) did include the fat pad deloading technique in conjunction with the patellar taping technique in a randomised controlled trial (RCT) on patellofemoral OA, but only reported on the effect of tape on the patella lateral transition and lateral tilt (Level II).
- McConnell (2000) reported the use of this technique to unload the fat pad in a case report (Clinical report).

Material

- Hypoallergenic underlay 3×15–20 cm strips.
- Rigid tape 3×10–15 cm strips.

Patient position

- Supine with knee resting on a rolled towel in approximately 20–$30°$ knee flexion.

Therapist position

- Standing beside the patient.

51

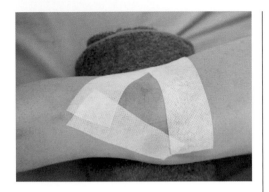 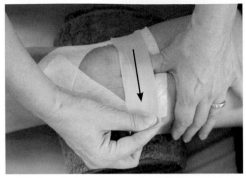 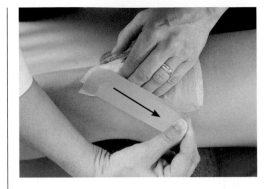

1 Apply hypoallergenic underlay superior to the patella.

2 Apply two strips of hypoallergenic underlay in an oblique direction from the tibial tuberosity medially and laterally towards the knee joint line, to meet the superior strip of hypoallergenic underlay. The combined effect of the hypoallergenic underlay strips should appear as a triangle shape around the patella.

3 Apply a strip of tape superior to the patella with one hand while applying pressure to tilt the patella anteriorly with the other hand — this lifts the patella inferior pole off the fat pad. Apply the tape from lateral to medial.

4 Apply a strip of tape medially from the tibial tuberosity and, while tensioning the tape with one hand, gather the tissues and lift towards the centre of the patella, further unloading the patella off the fat pad.

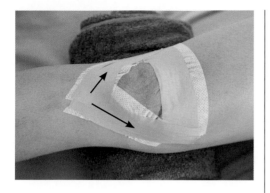

5 Repeat step 4 on the lateral aspect. This should result in a puckered appearance of the soft tissues around the patella.

6 Support the tape on each side of the knee using the therapist's hands and ask the patient to actively flex the knee, while ensuring the tape adheres during the movement laterally and medially. This will enhance the tape adhesion.

Reassessment
○ Comfort and symptoms at rest.
○ Patient's provocative movement(s) and symptoms.

51

Chondromalacia patella

Background and rationale

Chondromalacia patella is one of the conditions that can cause PFPS. It is associated with erosion or changes of the chondral retropatella surface. Pain and functional limitations associated with chondomalacia patella or PFPS may be improved using a therapeutic treatment program first described by Jenny McConnell (1986). Using tape to unload the patella as an adjunct to usual management may prove beneficial in providing pain relief associated with the patella rubbing against the trochlea during movement. This technique is similar to the technique described for patella fat pad deloading in the previous section, however the tape is applied closer to the patella and the patella and soft tissues are gathered and lifted upwards towards the centre of the tape triangle.

Evidence

○ No research studies relating to this technique were identified.

Material

○ Hypoallergenic underlay 3 × 15–20 cm strips.
○ Rigid tape 3 × 10–15 cm strips.

Patient position

○ Supine with knee resting on a rolled towel in approximately 20–30° knee flexion.

Therapist position

○ Standing beside the patient.

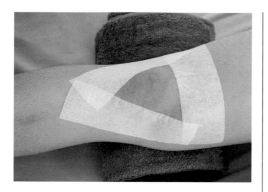

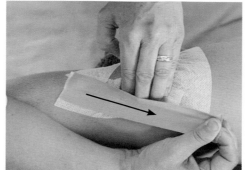

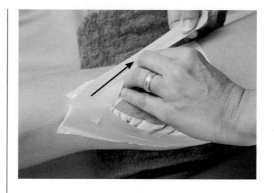

1   Apply hypoallergenic underlay superior to the patella.

2   Apply two strips of hypoallergenic underlay in an oblique direction from the tibial tuberosity medially and laterally towards the knee joint line, to meet the superior strip of hypoallergenic underlay. The combined effect of the hypoallergenic underlay strips should appear as a triangle shape around the patella.

3   Apply a strip of tape medially from the tibial tuberosity close to the patella border and while tensioning the tape with one hand gather the tissues and lift towards the centre of the patella, further unloading the patella off the trochlea with the other hand.

4   Repeat step 4 on the lateral aspect.

52

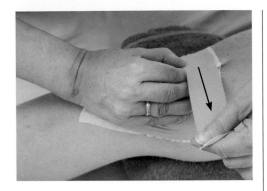 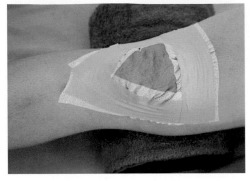

5 Apply a strip of tape superior and lateral to the patella close to the patella superior border and while tensioning the tape with one hand gather the tissues and lift towards the centre of the patella, further unloading the patella off the trochlea with the other hand.

6 Support the tape on each side of the knee using the therapist's hands and ask patient to actively flex the knee, while ensuring the tape adheres during the movement laterally and medially. This will enhance the tape adhesion.

Reassessment

○ Comfort and symptoms at rest.
○ Patient's provocative movement(s) and symptoms.

52

Patella tendon deloading

Background and rationale

Patellar tendinopathy is a continuum of pathological changes and may be associated with degeneration of the patellar tendon. The patient may present with anterior knee pain aggravated by jumping, hopping or bouncing (Brukner & Khan 2007). Other activities that load the patella tendon, particularly during eccentric knee flexion in weight bearing, may also aggravate the symptoms. Management of the condition is complex and can include eccentric exercises, load modification, a focus on improving the shock-absorbing capacity of the limb and addressing the musculotendinous pathology (Cook et al 2001). Tape used as an adjunct to usual management may provide additional symptom relief. This taping technique's proposed effect is to unload the patellar tendon thus reducing the symptoms during quadriceps muscle contraction. Unloading the patellar tendon with tape, particularly at the insertion on the tibial tubersosity, may also be beneficial in young athletes with Osgood Schlatter's Disease.

A variety of patella tendon straps are widely available on the market and many therapists may prescribe them in the management of patellar tendon conditions. Although it is not our aim to discuss the use of patella straps in this book, patella straps were found to reduce the patellofemoral contact area and pressure as well as reduce the pressure on the infrapatellar structures in a cadaveric study (Bohnsack et al 2008). This taping technique may resemble the patella tendon strap and may be used in a similar manner in the absence of patella tendon straps.

Evidence

○ No research studies relating to this technique were identified.

Material

○ Hypoallergenic underlay 1 × 10–15 cm strip.
○ Rigid tape 1 × 10 cm and 1 × 15 cm strips.

Patient position

○ Supine with knee resting on a rolled towel in approximately 20–30° knee flexion.

Therapist position

○ Standing beside the patient.

53

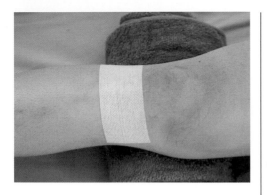

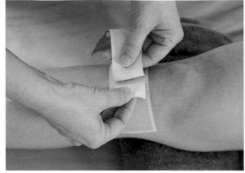

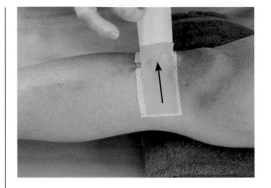

1 Apply hypoallergenic underlay horizontally over the patellar tendon.

2 Apply the two strips of tape 5–8 cm on either side of the patellar tendon, placing the longer strip of tape on the lateral side.

3 Join and press the two strips of tape together over the centre of the patellar tendon, and traction the tape upwards, lifting the tendon up.

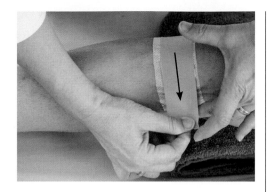

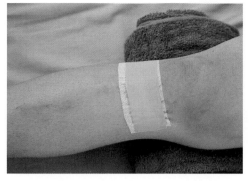

4 With one hand gather the medial tissues of the knee while with the other hand tensioning the longer strip of tape and applying it on the medial aspect of the knee.

5 Support the tape on each side of the knee using the therapist's hands and ask the patient to actively flex the knee, while ensuring the tape adheres during the movement laterally and medially. This will enhance the tape adhesion.

Reassessment
○ Comfort and symptoms at rest.
○ Patient's provocative movement(s) and symptoms.

53

Superior and inferior tibiofibular joints

Superior tibiofibular joint subluxation

Background and rationale

Dislocation of the superior tibiofibular joint is an uncommon injury that is usually classified into types I–IV: I subluxation, II antero-lateral dislocation (most common), III postero-medial dislocation, and IV superior dislocation (Harvey & Woods 1992). A number of cases have been reported, some of which are associated with fibular fractures (Herscovici et al 1992; Gabrion et al 2003). In type I injuries that are associated with subluxation of the fibular head, tape may be used as an adjunct to usual management. Brian Mulligan first mentioned taping the superior tibiofibular joint after mobilisation with movement (MWM) techniques proposing it keeps the 'fibula head in position' (Mulligan 1999). The patient's symptom response to taping needs to be assessed to ascertain the benefit of the technique. The taping direction will depend on which direction the subluxation has occurred, anterior or posterior, and which direction of the MWM the patient has responded to the most.

Evidence

○ No research studies relating to this technique were identified.

Material

○ Hypoallergenic underlay 1 × 15 cm strip.
○ Rigid tape 1 × 15 cm strip.

Patient position

○ Supine with knee in 90° knee flexion.

Therapist position

○ Standing beside the patient.

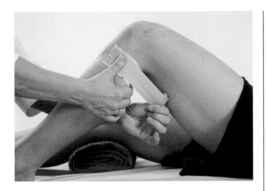
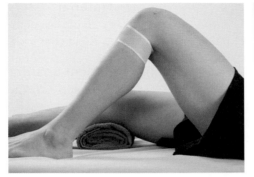

1 Apply hypoallergenic underlay horizontally over the fibula head, extending it approximately 5 cm each way of the anterior posterior borders of the fibula head.

2 Apply an antero-posterior or a postero-anterior glide on the symptomatic side either as an accessory glide, as described by Maitland (2005) and compare which is hypo-mobile, or as an MWM as described in Mulligan (1999) and decide which direction provides symptom relief.

3 For an antero-posterior glide apply the tape anterior or posterior to the fibula head, tension the tape with one hand and apply an anterior or posterior glide on the fibula head as the tape is placed over the joint.

4 For a postero-anterior glide apply the tape posterior to the fibula head, tension the tape with one hand and apply a posterior glide on the fibula head as tape is placed over the joint.

Reassessment
○ Position of fibula head with patient in supine position and knee flexed to 90°.
○ Comfort and symptoms at rest.
○ Patient's provocative movement(s) and symptoms.

54

Inferior tibiofibular joint subluxation

Background and rationale

Inferior tibiofibular (tib–fib) joint subluxation is purported to occur in some lateral ankle sprains leading to a fibular 'positional fault' (Kavanagh 1999; Hubbard & Hertel 2008). Brian Mulligan first mentioned the use of mobilisation with movement (MWM) manual therapy techniques on the inferior tib–fib joint as a treatment approach to recalcitrant inversion ankle sprains (Mulligan 1999). Mulligan proposes that injury to the lateral ligaments in ankle sprain may cause the fibula to translate anteriorly. He uses an antero-posterior cranial glide on the inferior fibula with active inversion as an MWM, which he proposes can decrease symptoms of pain and swelling (Mulligan 1999). Tape is used post MWM to 'hold the fibula in place' (Mulligan 1999). Mulligan's concept was first tested in a single case study by O'Brien and Vicenzino (1998) and the authors showed that using MWMs of the inferior tib–fib joint superimposed with tape showed greater improvement in pain, function and ankle ROM.

Evidence

○ A single case study by O'Brien and Vicenzino (1998) did find that MWM and tape were beneficial in improving pain, function and ankle ROM post lateral ankle sprain (Level IV).
○ A pilot study by Moiler et al (2006) found the use of this technique was effective in prevention of ankle sprains in individuals with and without history of previous ankle sprain compared to a different form of ankle prophylaxis (Level III-3).

Material

○ Hypoallergenic underlay 1 × 15 cm strip (optional).
○ Rigid tape 1 × 15 cm strip.

Patient position

○ Supine with knee in extension and the foot over the edge of the bed.

Therapist position

○ Sitting or standing at the end of the bed, near the patient's foot.

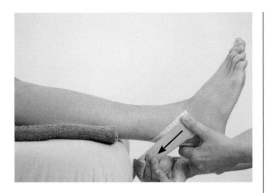

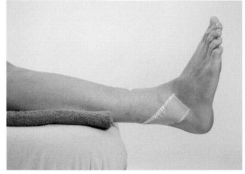

1   Apply hypoallergenic underlay in an antero-postero-cranial direction over the inferior tib–fib joint 1 cm anterior to the edge of the fibula and 1 cm from the distal end of the fibula and direct the tape posteriorly in an oblique direction slightly above the tendo-Achilles. Finish the hypoallergenic underlay antero-medially well above the medial malleolus.

2   Apply tape over the inferior tib–fib joint, tension the tape with one hand and apply it in an oblique cranial direction over the hypoallergenic underlay, while applying an antero-posterior cranial glide on the fibula with the other hand.

3   Direct the tape posteriorly slightly above the tendo-Achilles and finish the tape antero-medially.

4   It is possible to apply a second strip of tape over the first one repeating step 2, but this is optional.

Reassessment

○ Comfort and symptoms at rest.

○ Active ankle ROM and associated pain using VAS.

○ Patient's provocative activity such as gait and symptoms.

55

Ankle joint

Basket weave

Background and rationale

Ankle sprains are very common, particularly in sporting activities (Beynnon et al 2005; Ivins 2006; Fong et al 2008). Management of acute ankle sprains will usually involve ice, compression, elevation and early guided functional mobilisation with relative rest (Herrington & Al-Shammari 2006; Ivins 2006). A number of ankle sprains may lead to recurrence with chronic instability of the ankle joint (Hubbard & Hicks-Little 2008). Tape may be used as an adjunct to usual management in acute, subacute and chronic ankle sprains and can be used to target oedema, provide support, restrict extreme ranges, increase proprioception and prevent recurrence (Arnold & Docherty 2004). In chronic ankle sprains where ongoing support may be required a brace may be more cost effective (Olmsted et al 2004). However, tape may be used in the interim or in the absence of a brace.

The basket weave taping technique encompasses the entire ankle. It uses: anchors around the ankle; stirrups (tape in a longitudinal direction going under the foot from medial to lateral direction, simulating the stirrup in a horse's saddle); spurs (tape in horizontal direction going behind the heel in a lateral to medial direction, simulating the heel spurs on cowboy boots); reverse sixes (tape starting on the lower end of the 6 and finishing on the upper end of the 6); sixes (tape starting on the upper end of the 6 and finishing on the lower end of the 6); a heel lock (figure-8 tape around the heel and the sole of the foot); and lock-offs (locking strips of tape superimposing the tape ends of the stirrups, reverse

6s and 6s). The origin of this technique and further information regarding its development is described in Chapter 2 (p 10).

This technique is not usually performed in the first 48 hours after an injury where severely increasing swelling is present, but rather once the rate of swelling increase has slowed down. Instead, in acute ankle sprains where severe swelling is present an open basket weave technique may be performed. This involves leaving the anterior aspect of the foot and ankle open with the tape not connected together, to allow the swelling to expand without causing a constriction that may compromise the circulation. This technique is described in the next section on page 170.

Evidence

○ Research in this area uses varied techniques and mostly relates to injury prevention rather than injury management.

○ A study by Rarick et al (1962) compared different taping techniques for the ankle and found that the basket weave with stirrups and heel lock was more supportive than the normal basket weave with no heel lock. However, the authors concluded that up to 40% of the support was lost after 10 minutes of vigorous exercise (Level IV).

○ A comparative radiological study was conducted by Vaes et al (1985) to evaluate the effectiveness of the closed basket weave taping technique with no heel lock. They found that the basket weave was superior to elastic adhesive bandage in resisting talar tilt when an inversion force was applied (Level IV).

○ No other recent studies that directly compared the effect of basket weave with another ankle taping technique were identified.

Material

○ Approximately half a roll of rigid tape. Strips of tape will need to be torn off the roll as the technique is being applied, based on measurement of the patient's foot. There will be approximately:
  • 7–10 × 35–50 cm stirrups, 6s and reverse 6s strips
  • 6–8 × 35–50 cm spur strips
  • 4–5 × 20–30 cm strips for an anchor and lock-offs
  • 1 × 80–100 cm strip for the heel lock.

○ Foam under-wrap may be used under the tape if the patient is sensitive to tape (optional).

○ A small piece of high-density foam in the shape of a U may be applied around the malleoli if there is oedema present around the area (optional).

Patient position

○ Supine with the foot resting over the edge of the bed.

○ The foot is in plantigrade position with neutral eversion/inversion.

Therapist position

○ Sitting or standing at the end of the bed, near the patient's foot.

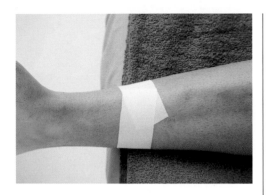

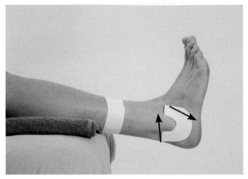

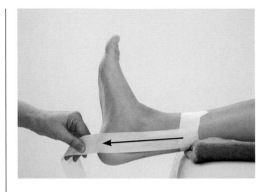

1   Apply a superior anchor on the leg, 4–5 cm above the malleoli, joining the anchor ends obliquely on the anterior aspect of the lower leg.

2   The small piece of high-density foam may be applied around the lateral and/or medial malleolus now if it will be included in the technique.

3   Apply a stirrup medial to lateral, starting on the anchor medio-posteriorly, directing the tensioned tape behind the medial malleolus, under the foot in a medial to lateral direction and finishing the tape behind the lateral malleolus on the postero-lateral aspect of the anchor.

56

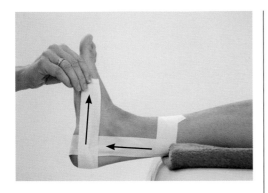

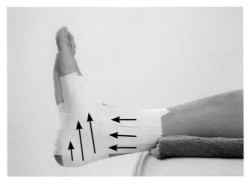

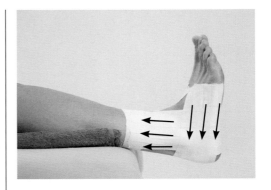

4 Apply a heel spur starting along the fifth metatarsal (MT), directing the tape posterior to the calcaneum laterally to medially and finishing the tape along the first MT.

5 Repeat alternating stirrups and heel spurs (approximately 4–5 strips of each), ensuring overlap of each previous layer with half the width of the new layer. The interlaced strips of tape will form a basket weave effect, hence the name 'basket weave'.

6 Once the tape has reached just anterior to the ankle, strips of tape in reverse 6 and 6 can be used in place of stirrups, which by locking the tape on itself as occurs when using these types of taping technique will add to the stability effect of the tape.

56

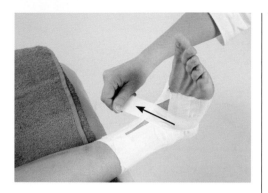 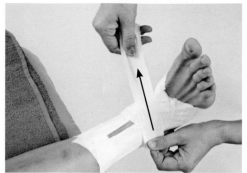 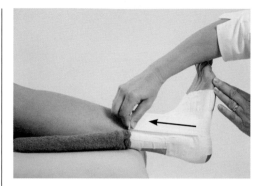

7 The 6s start on the medial aspect of the anchor and are applied in a medial to lateral direction in the same way as the stirrups; however, when the tape reaches the lateral ankle it is directed over the dorsum of the foot, locking on itself near the medial malleolus.

8 The reverse 6s start on the lateral malleolus, and are directed over the dorsum of the foot from lateral to medial and under the plantar aspect of the foot from medial to lateral, overlapping the starting tape end of the reverse 6 (locking it in place) and finishing on the lateral aspect of the anchor.

9 There will be approximately two reverse 6s and two 6s depending on the size of the patient's foot.

10 Continue to alternate each reverse 6 and each 6 with an ascending spur around the lower leg. Once you have reached the superior anchor with the spurs, it should create the basket weaving effect.

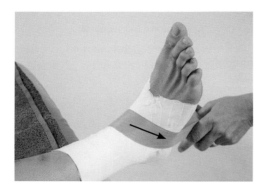

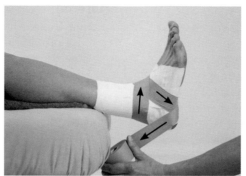

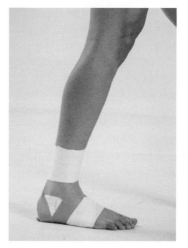

11 Apply a full heel lock with a single piece of tape.
  • Start the tape on the medial malleolus.
  • Bring the tape anteriorly over the anterior ankle joint line to below the lateral malleolus.
  • Continue the tape under the plantar surface of the foot from lateral to medial.
  • Next, cross the medial aspect of the calcanium obliquely across the posterior calcaneum then across the lateral malleolus to the anteriour ankle joint line.
  • Continue medially under the plantar aspect of the foot, medial to lateral, and cross the lateral calcaneum obliquely.
  • Continue posteriorly around the posterior calcaneum and finish on the tape that is already in place on the anteriour ankle joint line.

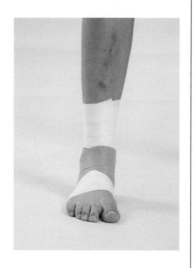

12 Apply 4–5 lock-offs over the stirrups. Ensure there is no exposed skin for oedema to move into.

Reassessment
○ Circulation, patient comfort and symptoms at rest.
○ Passive and active available ROM and symptoms.
○ Provocative activity, such as gait and symptoms.

Open basket weave

Background and rationale

As discussed in the section above, in acute ankle sprains where severe oedema is present an open basket weave technique is advised. The anterior aspect of the taping technique on the dorsum of the foot remains open, with the tape ends not connected together. This technique provides some support and compression to the oedematous lateral and medial ankle while allowing room for the expanding oedema. It may be a useful technique in the first 48 hours of acute ankle sprains as an adjunct to usual first aid and physiotherapy management.

The open basket weave taping technique only uses an anchor around the fibula and tibia high above the malleoli (which can remain open), stirrups, spurs and open lock-offs (the description of these terms is outlined in the basket weave ankle taping technique in the previous section).

Evidence

○ No research studies relating to this technique were identified.

Material

○ Approximately half a roll of rigid tape. Strips of tape will need to be torn off the roll as the technique is being applied, based on measurement of the patient's foot. There will be approximately:
  • 7–20 × 35–50 cm stirrup strips
  • 6–8 × 35–50 cm spur strips
  • 4 × 20–30 cm strips for an anchor and lock-offs.
○ A small piece of high-density foam in the shape of a U may be applied around the malleoli (optional).

Patient position

○ Supine with the foot resting over the edge of the bed.
○ The foot is in plantigrade position and neutral eversion/inversion.

Therapist position

○ Sitting or standing at the end of the bed, near the patient's foot.

57

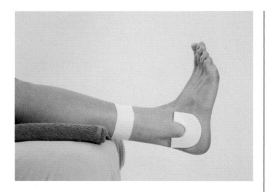 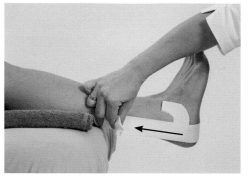 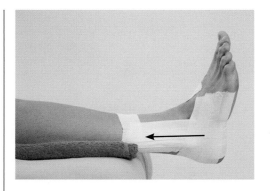

1 Apply a superior anchor on the leg, 5–10 cm above the malleoli, preferably leaving the anchor ends open on the anterior aspect of the lower leg.

2 A small piece of high-density foam may be applied around the lateral and/or medial malleolus now if it will be included in the technique.

3 Apply a stirrup medial to lateral, starting on the anchor medio-posteriorly, directing the tensioned tape behind the medial malleolus, under the foot in a medial to lateral direction and finishing the tape behind the lateral malleolus on the postero-lateral aspect of the anchor.

4 Apply a heel spur starting along the fifth metatarsal (MT), directing the tape posterior to the calcaneum laterally to medially and finishing the tape along the first MT.

5 Repeat alternating stirrups and heel spurs (approximately 4–5 strips of each), ensuring overlap of each previous layer with half the width of the new layer. The interlaced strips of tape will form a basket weave effect, hence the name 'basket weave'.

57

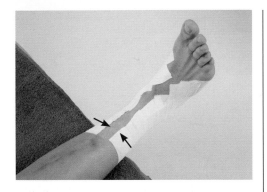

6   Apply 4–5 open lock-offs (tape ends
    not connected anteriorly on the ankle)
    over the stirrups.
7   For injuries where oedema is an issue,
    an elasticised support bandage worn
    over the taping technique is
    sometimes advised.

Reassessment

○   Circulation, patient comfort and
    symptoms at rest.
○   Passive and active available ROM and
    symptoms.
○   Provocative activity and symptoms.

57

Ankle anti-inversion

Background and rationale

During the rehabilitation phase of ankle sprains, as the patient is not requiring maximum compression for oedema and support, a technique using fewer stirrups, no spurs, 2 × reverse 6s, 2 × 6s, a heel lock and lock-offs may be useful (a description of these terms is outlined previously, technique 56). This technique may be used by athletes returning to sports after an injury or by athletes who have not sustained an injury but wish to tape their ankles prophylactically, as is the requirement in certain sports.

The anti-inversion taping technique can be adapted and used as an anti-eversion technique in patients with deltoid ligament sprain. The direction of the stirrups is reversed so the stirrups will start laterally and are directed medially, to provide support to the medial structures.

Evidence

- No research studies relating to this technique were identified.
- Research in this area uses varied techniques and mostly relates to injury prevention rather than injury management.
- Tape applied at the ankle with stirrups resists inversion (Vaes et al 1985) (Level IV).

Material

- Approximately half a roll of rigid tape. Strips of tape will need to be torn off the roll as the technique is being applied, based on measurement of the patient's foot. There will be approximately:
  - 7–10 × 35–50 cm stirrups, 6s and reverse 6s strips
  - 4–5 × 20–30 cm strips for an anchor and lock-offs
  - 1 × 80–100 cm strip for the heel lock.
- Foam under-wrap may be used under the tape if the patient is sensitive to tape (optional).
- A small piece of high-density foam in the shape of a U may be applied around the malleoli if there is oedema present around the area (optional).

Patient position

- Supine with the foot resting over the edge of the bed.
- The foot is in plantigrade position and neutral eversion/inversion.

Therapist position

- Sitting or standing at the end of the bed, near the patient's foot.

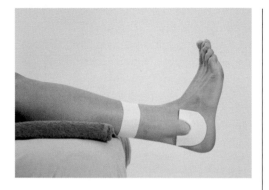

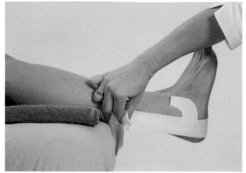

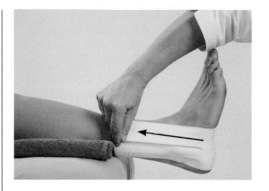

1 Apply a superior anchor on the leg, 4–5 cm above the malleoli, joining the anchor ends obliquely on the anterior aspect of the lower leg.

2 A small piece of high-density foam may be applied around the lateral and/or medial malleolus now if it will be included in the technique.

3 Apply a stirrup medial to lateral, starting on the anchor medio-posteriorly, directing the tensioned tape behind the medial malleolus, under the foot in a medial to lateral direction and finishing the tape behind the lateral malleolus on the postero-lateral aspect of the anchor.

4 Repeat step 2 with two more stirrups, moving from posterior to anterior direction overlapping each previous stirrup with half the width of the new strip of tape. Ensure the medial and lateral malleoli are covered.

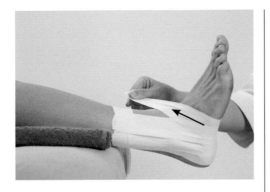
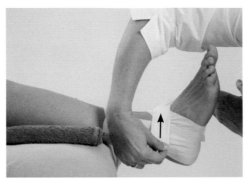
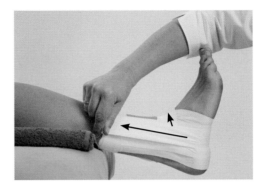

5 Apply two 6s overlapping each one by half the tape width of the previous one. The 6s start on the medial aspect of the anchor, are applied in a medial to lateral direction in the same way as the stirrups, however, when the tape reaches the lateral ankle it is directed over the dorsum of the foot, locking on itself near the medial malleolus.

6 Apply two reverse 6s overlapping each one by half the tape width of the previous one. The reverse 6s start on the lateral malleolus, are directed over the dorsum of the foot from lateral to medial and under the plantar aspect of the foot from medial to lateral, overlap the starting tape end of the reverse 6 (locking it in place) and finish on the lateral aspect of the anchor.

58

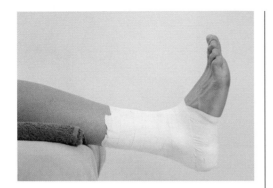

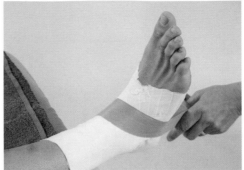

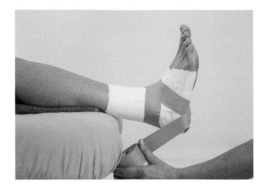

The application of a heel lock is described in the following images:

7 Apply a full heel lock with a single piece of tape.
  • Start the tape on the medial malleolus.
  • Bring the tape anteriorly over the anterior ankle joint line to below the lateral malleolus.
  • Continue the tape under the plantar surface of the foot from lateral to medial.
  • Next, cross the medial aspect of the calcanium obliquely across the posterior calcaneum then across the lateral malleolus to the anteriour ankle joint line.
  • Continue medially under the plantar aspect of the foot, medial to lateral, and cross the lateral calcaneum obliquely.

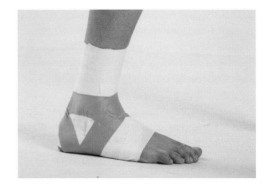

  • Continue posteriorly around the posterior calcaneum and finish on the tape that is already in place on the anteriour ankle joint line.
8 Apply 4–5 lock-offs over the stirrups. Ensure there is no exposed skin within the tape strips.

58

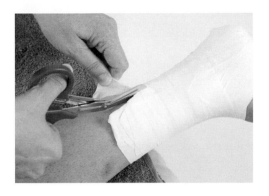
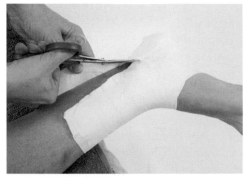

Removing the basket weave and anti-inversion

1   It is best to remove the tape using blunt nose scissors. The starting position is on the medial aspect of the ankle, in line with immediately posterior to the medial malleolus.

2   Proceed to cut through the thick layers of tape with the scissors, folding the tape back as moving posterior to the medial malleolus.

Reassessment

○ Circulation, patient comfort and symptoms at rest.

○ Passive and active available ROM and symptoms.

○ Provocative activity, such as gait and symptoms.

58

Triceps surae and/or Achilles tendon complex

Background and rationale

Conditions affecting the triceps surae and/or Achilles tendon complex include muscle and tendon strains or tendinopathy. Management can include a heel raise to reduce tensile strain on the complex, especially for muscle strains (Brukner & Khan 2007). Taping the foot into a plantarflexed position can mimic the effect of a heel raise to reduce strain on torn or vulnerable tissues, especially in the acute phase or during vigorous activity such as sport. However, the therapist should bear in mind that for Achilles tendinopathy conditions eccentric muscle training has been found to be an effective treatment (Woodley et al 2007). It is thus recommended that taping into a shortened position is only applied for short periods of time when tensile forces on the complex are likely to be high, such as during sporting competition.

This technique may be applied post triceps surae muscle injury or strain in the acute and subacute phases to reduce passive and active dorsiflexion ROM. By decreasing the passive and active dorsiflexion ROM the injured muscle fibres may experience less provocation into pain and disability.

Evidence

○ No research studies relating to this technique were identified.

Material

○ Rigid tape 1 × 60–80 cm strip (depending on the height of the patient).
○ Rigid tape 2 × 30–40 cm strips for anchor and lock-off.
○ Rigid tape 60 cm strips for optional reinforcements.

Patient position

○ Prone, with the foot over the edge of the bed.
○ The foot is in slight plantarflexed position.

Therapist position

○ Standing at the foot of the bed, near the patient's foot.

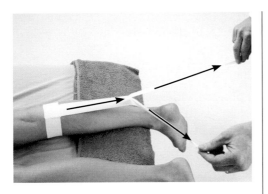

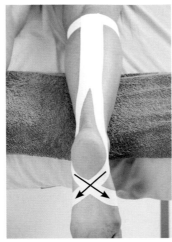

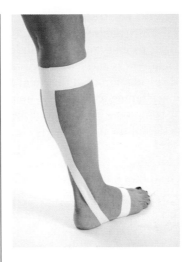

1 Apply an anchor around the superior leg, above the triceps surae muscle belly.
2 Apply the long strip of tape from the anchor above the muscle belly of the triceps surae muscle in a longitudinal direction.
3 At the point where the Achilles tendon becomes prominent to the end of the non-adhered tape, tear the tape longitudinally in half.
4 Apply one end of the torn tape towards the lateral aspect of the calcaneum and around the dorsal aspect of the foot.

5 Apply the other end of torn tape towards the medial aspect of the foot and around the dorsum of the foot joining it to the first end of the torn tape (simulate a figure 8).
6 Reinforcing strips can be applied over the dorsum of the foot and around the lateral and medial aspects of the calcaneum (optional).

7 Apply a lock-off over the anchor to secure the longitudinal tape.
8 For injuries where oedema is an issue, an elasticised support bandage worn over the taping technique is sometimes preferred.

Reassessment
○ Circulation, patient comfort and symptoms at rest.
○ Passive and active available ROM and symptoms.
○ Provocative activity and symptoms.

59

Shin deloading

Background and rationale

In medial tibial stress syndrome (MTSS) or shin splints as is the common term the usual symptoms include pain during activity and localised tenderness at the posterior tibial border resulting from the overload adaptation of the tibial cortex (Moen et al 2009). Applying a taping technique to unload the painful area and relieve the symptoms may assist in the recovery and/or increased function of the patient.

Evidence

○ No research studies relating to this technique were identified.

Material

○ Hypoallergenic underlay 2 × 5–10 cm strips.
○ Rigid tape 2 × 5–10 cm strips.

Patient position

○ Supine or long sitting position with knee resting on a rolled towel.

Therapist position

○ Standing beside the patient on the side to be taped.

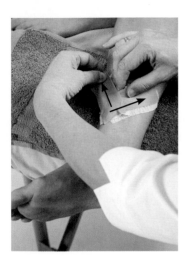

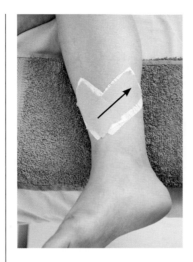

1 Identify and mark the area of tenderness over the medial tibial border.

2 Apply two strips of hypoallergenic underlay inferior to the tender area, one strip from lateral to medial, and one strip from medial to lateral direction forming a 'V' shape around the tenderness.

3 Apply a tensioned strip of tape inferior to the tender area towards the lateral superior direction with one hand, while the other hand is around the tender tissues lifting and gathering them towards the centre of the 'V'.

4 Apply a second strip of tape inferior to the tender area towards the medial superior direction with one hand while the other hand is around the tender tissues lifting and gathering them towards the centre of the 'V'.

5 The finished tape should look like a 'V' around the tender shin area.

Reassessment
○ Comfort and symptoms at rest.
○ Provocative movement, functional tasks and symptoms.

60

Foot

Anti-pronation – low dye, augmented low dye and plantar fasciitis low dye

Background and rationale

Abnormal foot pronation has been reported in the literature to be associated with lower limb conditions (Moen et al 2009). Management of abnormal foot pronation can include the use of orthotics. Taping to reduce abnormal pronation can be used as a temporary measure to evaluate the likely benefit of orthotics (Vicenzino 2004) and as a therapeutic tool in the management of these conditions.

The most common anti-pronation taping techniques frequently used by therapists and studied in the literature are the low dye and augmented low dye (Vicenzino et al 2000; Vicenzino 2004; Vicenzino et al 2005). These techniques aim to maintain the medial longitudinal arch height during the stance phase of walking and running, with augmented low dye being shown to be superior to low dye (Vicenzino et al 2005).

There is good evidence to support the efficacy of the low dye taping techniques to reduce abnormal foot pronation, with details of the proposed effects being further explored in Chapter 2.

As one example, plantar fasciitis or fasciopathy is a condition commonly associated with plantar heel pain and excessive or prolonged foot pronation, with altered function of the windlass mechanism (Jamali et al 2004). The patient may experience symptoms of pain on weight bearing and during walking which could limit them from participating in normal activities of daily living. Management of plantar fasciitis may include manual therapy, exercise, electrophysical modalities (Cleland et al 2009) and taping. Taping that reduces abnormal foot pronation and maintains the height of the medial longitudinal arch (MLA) may also reduce strain on the plantar fascia, thereby reducing pain associated with plantar fasciitis (Jamali et al 2004; O'Sullivan et al 2008). The low dye taping techniques described in the following section may be a useful adjunct to other treatment modalities for this condition. Specifically, a taping technique that incorporates the low dye anti-pronation taping procedure, with 1–2 plantar fascia strips applied on the plantar surface of the foot prior to the application of mini stirrups, may be a beneficial adaptation of the techniques and it is the third of the three techniques further described here.

The following three techniques incorporate the use of low dye either as a stand-alone technique, with added augmentation or with the use of half figure 8s over the plantar fascia for patients with plantar fasciitis.

Low dye

Evidence

- Augmented low dye taping is superior to low dye for increasing MLA height (Vicenzino et al 2005).
- Low dye taping reduces strain on the plantar fascia (Bartold et al 2009).

Material

- Rigid tape 2 × 35–40 cm strips.
- Rigid tape 5–6 × 15–20 cm strips (depending on the length of the patient's foot).
- Rigid tape 1 × 15–20 cm strip to lock-off superiorly.

Patient position

- Supine or long sitting on the bed, with the foot over the edge, subtalar joint neutral position, with slight supination at the mid-foot.

Therapist position

- Sitting or standing at the edge of the foot of the bed.

Procedure

(as adapted from Vicenzino et al 2005)

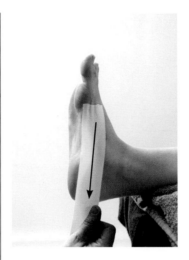

1 Apply a heel spur starting medially and proximal to first metatarsophalangeal (MTP) joint to encourage forefoot adduction and plantar flexion of the first ray, and directing the tape posterior to the calcaneum laterally to finish at the base of the fifth MTP joint.

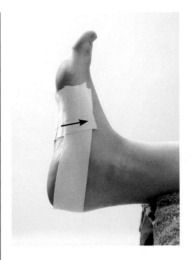

2 Apply mini stirrups perpendicular to the foot, from lateral aspect of the spur directing them medially under the plantar surface of the foot, finishing on the medial aspect of the spur. Ensure not to wrinkle the plantar skin of the foot or the mini stirrups.

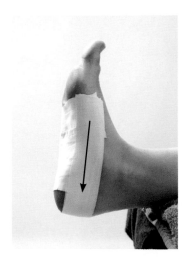

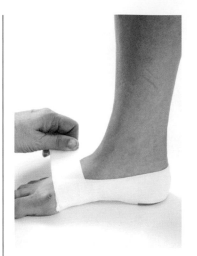

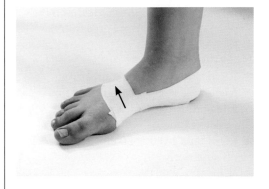

3 The mini lateral to medial stirrups start under the metatarsal heads, leaving the MTP joints free, and then move posteriorly towards the sustentaculum talus. Ensure the mini stirrups only overlap by half the width of the tape. As the mini stirrups are applied the plantar arch and the navicular tuberosity are supported.

4 Apply a second heel spur medial to lateral over the same direction as the first one as a lock-off.

5 Stand the patient up and check for comfort. Apply a lock-off strip of tape on the dorsum of the foot, over the metatarsal head, joining the calcaneal lock-off spur from medial to lateral.

Reassessment

○ Circulation, comfort and symptoms at rest and in static standing.
○ Vertical navicular height.
○ Gait and/or running — biomechanical and/or symptom changes.

Augmented low dye

Evidence
○ Augmented low dye increased medial longitudinal arch height and reduced EMG activity of tibialis anterior and tibialis posterior muscles during walking (Franettovich et al 2008).
○ Augmented low dye taping is superior to low dye for increasing MLA height (Vicenzino et al 2005).

Material
○ Rigid tape 4 × 20–25 cm strips.
○ Rigid tape 2 × 50–60 cm strips.

Patient position
○ Supine or long sitting on the bed, with the foot over the edge, subtalar joint neutral position, with slight supination at the mid-foot.

Therapist position
○ Sitting or standing at the edge of the foot of the bed.

Procedure
(as adapted from Vicenzino et al 2005)

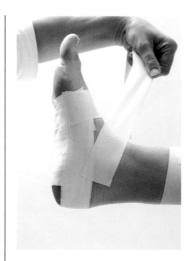

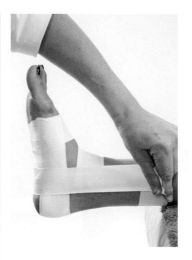

This taping is applied over the low dye taping described in technique 61.

1 Apply an anchor 10 cm above the malleoli (or one third above the length of the leg) with the ankle fully dorsiflexed, joining the two tape ends in an oblique orientation.

2 Apply the first 'reverse 6', starting on the medial malleolus directing it medial to lateral under the plantar surface of the mid-foot and supporting the navicular and the medial arch upwards.

3 At the medial malleolus cross the tape on itself and direct the posterior tape edge in line with the middle of the medial malleolus to finish medially on the anchor strip.

62

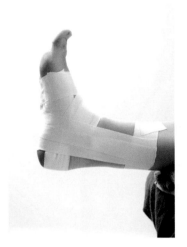

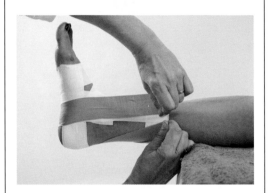

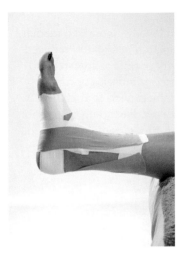

4 Repeat step 2 with a second 'reverse 6' tape in the same direction as the previous 'reverse 6', overlapping the previous strip of tape with half the tape width.

5 Repeat step 3, with a third 'reverse 6' ensuring the three 'reverse 6s' span from the middle of the medial malleolus proximally to cover the navicular distally.

6 Apply a calcaneal sling on the medial calcaneum, beginning anteriorly at the anchor and directing it obliquely under the plantar aspect of the mid-foot, posterior to the calcaneum and the malleolus and once again obliquely on the lateral aspect of the calcaneum aiming to finish it over the origin on the anchor strip.

7 Repeat step 5 with a second calcaneal sling, overlapping the first one.

8 Apply 3–4 lock-offs below the anchor, over the proximal insertions of the reverse 6s and the calcaneal slings.

Reassessment

○ Circulation, comfort and symptoms at rest and in static standing.

○ Vertical navicular height or medial longitudinal arch height using the McPoil et al method (McPoil et al 2008).

○ Gait and/or running– biomechanical and/or symptom changes.

Plantar fasciitis low dye

Evidence
- Augmented low dye taping is superior to low dye for increasing medial longitudinal arch (ML) height (Vicenzino et al 2005).
- Low dye taping reduces strain on the plantar fascia (Bartold et al 2009).
- A similar technique was found to significantly reduce pain in patients with plantar fasciitis (Jamali et al 2004).

Material
- Rigid tape 2 × 35–40 cm strips.
- Rigid tape 5–6 × 15–20 cm strips (depending on the length of the patient's foot).
- Rigid tape 2 × 40–50 cm strips for the plantar fascia support tape.
- Rigid tape 1 × 15–20 cm strip to lock-off superiorly.

Patient position
- Supine or long sitting on the bed, with the foot over the edge, subtalar joint neutral position, with slight supination at the mid-foot.

Therapist position
- Sitting or standing at the edge of the foot of the bed.

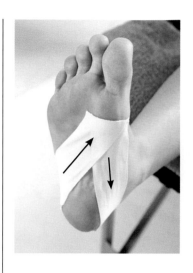
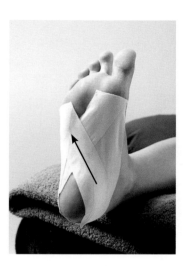

1 Apply a heel spur starting medially and proximal to first metatarsophalangeal (MTP) joint to encourage forefoot adduction and plantar flexion of the first ray. Direct the tape posterior to the calcaneum laterally to finish at the base of the fifth MTP joint.
2 Apply a tape strip in a half figure 8 on the plantar surface of the foot, starting at the first MTP and directing the tape on the medial border of the plantar surface posteriorly towards the calcaneum along the lateral border of the calcaneum and across the plantar aspect of the foot to finish the tape on the origin at the base of the first MTP.
3 Repeat with a second tape strip in a half figure 8 on the plantar surface of the foot, starting at the fifth MTP and directing the tape on the lateral border plantar surface posteriorly towards the calcaneum along the medial border of the calcaneum, across the foot to finish the tape on the origin at the base of the fifth MTP.

63

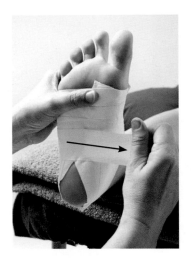 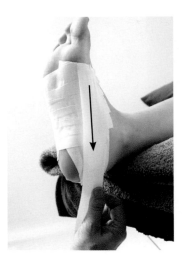

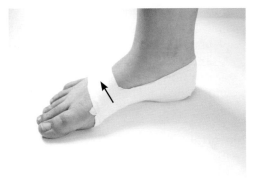

4 Apply mini stirrups perpendicular to the foot, from lateral aspect of the spur directing them medially under the plantar surface of the foot, finishing on the medial aspect of the spur. Ensure not to wrinkle the plantar skin of the foot or the mini stirrups.

5 The mini lateral to medial stirrups start under the metatarsal heads, leaving the MTP joints free, and then move posteriorly towards the sustentaculum talus. Ensure the mini stirrups only overlap by half the width of the tape. As the mini stirrups are applied the plantar arch and the navicular tuberosity are supported.

6 Apply a second heel spur medial to lateral over the same direction as the first one as a lock-off.

7 Stand patient up and check for comfort. Apply a lock-off strip of tape on the dorsum of the foot, over the metatarsal head, joining the calcaneal lock-off spur from medial to lateral.

Reassessment

○ Circulation, comfort and symptoms at rest and in standing.

○ Gait and/or running — biomechanical and/or symptom changes.

Heel fat pad deloading

Background and rationale

Pathology to the heel fat pad may be a cause of heel pain, which may lead to ongoing disability and inability to participate in normal activities such as walking. Management of heel pain may incorporate physiotherapy modalities such as manual therapy, exercise, electrotherapy (Cleland et al 2009) and taping.

This taping technique incorporates the use of mini stirrups under the heel to unload and support the painful heel fat pad.

Evidence

- No research studies relating to this technique were identified.

Material

- Rigid tape 1×15 cm strip.
- Rigid tape $4–5 \times 15–20$ cm strips.

Patient position

- Supine with the leg in extension and the foot resting on a towel over the end of the bed.

Therapist position

- Sitting or standing at the edge of the foot of the bed.

64

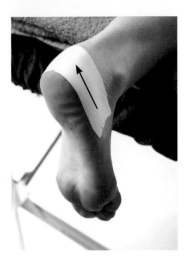

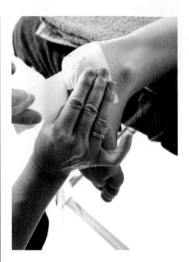

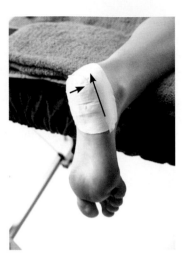

1 Apply a calcaneal spur from the lateral edge of the calcaneum at the calcaneocuboid junction to the medial edge of the calcaneum at the calcaneonavicular junction.

2 Apply a mini stirrup from medial plantar aspect of the heel (the calcaneum) and while tensioning the tape with one hand gather the fat pad tissues towards the middle of the heel with the other hand. Place the tape on the lateral aspect of the heel.

3 Repeat with a second mini stirrup, overlapping the previous one by half the width.

4 Repeat with a third and fourth mini stirrup, or as required based on the length of the patient's calcaneum.

5 Repeat step 1 with a calcaneal spur as a lock-off for the mini stirrups.

Reassessment

○ Circulation and symptoms at rest.
○ Provocative movement and symptoms.

64

Cuboid sling for cuboid syndrome

Background and rationale

Ongoing lateral and plantar mid-foot pain after a history of an ankle sprain may be indicative of cuboid syndrome (Jennings & Davies 2005) with possible bifurcate ligament trauma (Agnholt et al 1988). Thorough ankle and foot assessment which includes calcaneocuboid accessory glides and stress tests for the bifurcate ligament complex will assist in the diagnosis. Cuboid syndrome may involve a plantar or dorsal cuboid subluxation (Mooney & Maffey-Ward 1994), the direction usually being dependent on the initial mechanism of injury. Cuboid accessory glides in the opposite direction of the subluxation may provide immediate relief of pain and symptoms during walking. A cuboid manipulation may be performed by some therapists (Jennings & Davies 2005). As an adjunct to usual management of cuboid syndrome, a taping technique called cuboid sling can be used to support the cuboid, while concurrently maintaining a firm pressure in the direction of the relevant accessory glide (Mooney & Maffey-Ward 1994).

The following two therapeutic taping techniques address the plantar and dorsal directions of possible cuboid subluxations. They are very similar, but the starting positions and the direction the tape is coursed around the foot will depend on the directional subluxation of the cuboid. These techniques should be applied after careful assessment of the involvement of the cuboid.

Evidence

○ No research studies relating to this technique were identified.
○ Anecdotal evidence of the use of this technique (Jennings & Davies 2005, Mooney & Maffey-Ward 1994) (Clinical reports).
○ A case report on the use of taping for the treatment of cuboid syndrome was reported by Mazerolle (2007) (Clinical report).

Material

○ Rigid tape 1 × 15–20 cm strip.

Patient position

○ Supine with the leg in extension and the foot resting on a towel over the end of the bed.

Therapist position

○ Sitting or standing at the edge of the foot of the bed.

65

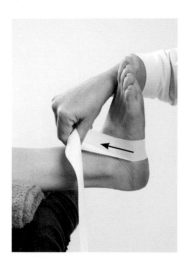

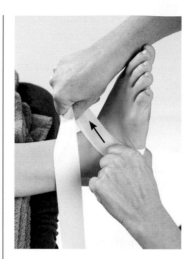

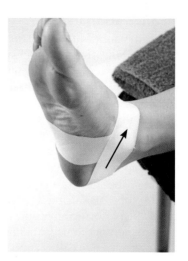

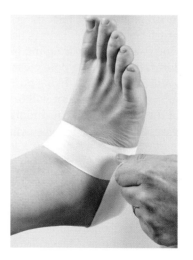

1 Start the tape on the medial aspect of the mid-foot, tension it and proceed under the plantar surface of the foot.

2 Direct the tape laterally over the dorsum of the cuboid towards the medial side, applying the tape with one hand as the cuboid is being glided into dorsal external rotation direction with the other hand.

3 Direct the tape over to lock-off the starting point of the tape, and continue posteriorly around the calcaneum from medial to lateral.

4 Finish the tape on the lateral side of the foot joining the tape strip over the cuboid.

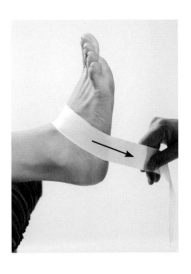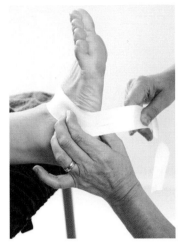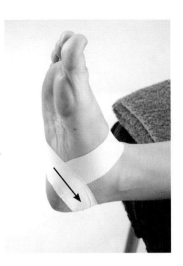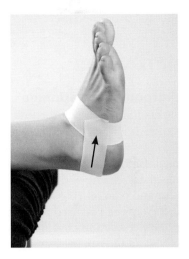

Cuboid plantar relocation for dorsal subluxation

1 Start the tape on the medial border of the foot over the navicular, tension it and direct the tape over the dorsum of the foot and dorsal surface of cuboid.
2 While tensioning the tape with one hand apply an accessory plantar and internal rotation glide on the cuboid with the other hand.
3 Direct the tape under the plantar surface of the foot to lock-off the origin of the tape over the navicular.
4 Proceed to direct the tape medially in a horizontal direction, posterior to the calcaneum from medial to lateral.
5 Finish the tape on the lateral side of the foot joining the tape strip over the cuboid.

Reassessment

○ Circulation and symptoms at rest.
○ Comfort — if this technique is applied too high on the dorsum of the foot the tape may interfere with dorsiflexion, so it is important to check for any discomfort dorsally at the ankle joint. If it is uncomfortable a small split can be made on half the width of the tape on its proximal edge. If it is still uncomfortable, then the tape needs to be removed and the taping procedure re-applied.
○ Passive and active ROM, provocative movement and symptoms.

65

Toe

Hallux valgus

Background and rationale

Various conditions affect the first metatarsophalangeal (MTP) joint such as hallux valgus, hallux limitus or rigidus and first MTP joint strain ('turf' toe). All of these conditions can result in pain and functional limitation. As an adjunct to usual management, taping of the first MTP may provide additional support and pain relief to the joint (Brukner & Khan 2007). Rigid or elastic tape can be used to protect the first MTP, including temporary correction of valgus deformity in hallux valgus, usually as an interim measure before orthotics are obtained.

This taping technique uses 19 mm strip of tape to reduce the valgus deformity of the hallux.

Evidence

○ No research studies relating to this technique were identified.

Material

○ Rigid tape 2 × 15 cm strips of tape for the anchor and lock-off.
○ Rigid tape 1 × 25 cm × 19 mm strip.
○ Rigid tape 1 × 10 cm × 19 mm strip.

Patient position

○ Supine, with the foot over the edge of the bed.

Therapist position

○ Standing or sitting on a chair at the end of the foot of the bed.

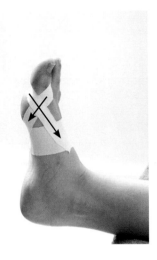

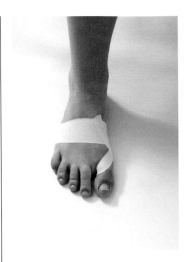

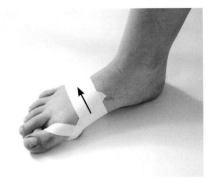

1. Apply a superior anchor on the first metatarsal (MT) on the medial border of the foot in a perpendicular direction.
2. Apply the centre of 25 cm × 19 mm wide tape strip on the lateral surface of the proximal first phalanx. Tension the two ends of the tape strip with each hand and apply a medial adduction glide to the proximal phalanx.

3. Cross the two ends of the tape strips over the medial border of the first MTP joint, forming a half 8.
4. Secure the tensioned tape strips to the anchor on the first MT on the medial border of the foot.
5. Apply a longitudinal tape strip from the proximal phalanx to the superior anchor (optional).

6. Place a lock-off tape strip over the superior anchor in a perpendicular direction to the foot.
7. Observe the corrected position of the first metatarsophalangeal joint.

Reassessment

○ Comfort, circulation and symptoms at rest.
○ Passive and active ROM, provocative movement and symptoms.

Toe interphalangeal joints

Background and rationale

Traumatic injuries to the foot and toes may result in symptoms of pain and stiffness with associated functional limitations. Clinical assessment of toes, which includes accessory joint glides, may reveal hypo-mobility associated with stiffness and/or painful motions at the metatarsophalangeal and/or interphalangeal joints (Maitland 2005). Rotational, transverse or antero-posterior accessory or mobilisation with movement (MWM) glides of the phalanges as part of treatment may provide symptom relief (Mulligan 1999). Tape may be used as a temporary adjunct to manual therapy and to usual management of toe injuries to provide a firm pressure on the involved phalanx, supporting the direction of the beneficial glide. Narrow elastic or rigid tape may be used.

Evidence

○ No research studies relating to this technique were identified.

Material

○ Rigid tape 1 × 15 cm × 19 mm strip.

Patient position

○ Patient is lying supine, with the foot over the edge of the treatment plinth.

Therapist position

○ Standing or sitting on a chair at the end of the foot of the bed.

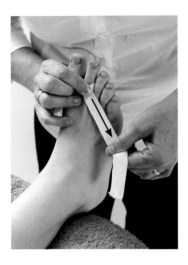

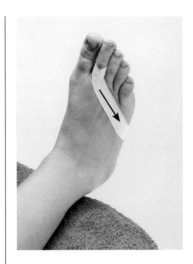

1 Identify the involved phalanx, provocative movement such as toe flexion or extension and the functional limitation, such as gait.

2 Identify the type and direction of glide to be used; transverse, rotation, postero-anterior or antero-posterior glide.

3 Perform the relevant accessory glide and ask patient to perform the provocative movement. If symptoms decrease tape may be beneficial.

4 Apply a narrow strip of tape on the affected phalanx, ensuring a firm pressure is directed towards the direction of the accessory glide.

5 Secure tape on the neighbouring phalanx or metatarsal of the involved toe.

Reassessment

○ Comfort, circulation and symptoms at rest.

○ Passive and active ROM, provocative movement and symptoms.

67

REFERENCES

Agnholt, J, Nielsen, S, Christensen, H (1988) Lesion of the ligamentum bifurcatum in ankle sprain. Arch Orthop Trauma Surg, 107(5): 326–8.

Arnold, B L, Docherty, C L (2004) Bracing and rehabilitation — what's new. Clinical Journal of Sport Medicine, 23(1): 83–95.

Bartold, S, Clarke, R, Franklyn-Miller, A, Falvey, E, Bryant, A, Briggs, C, McCrory, R (2009) The effect of taping on plantar fascia strain: a cadaveric study. Journal of Science and Medicine in Sport, 12 (suppl 1): S74–S75.

Bennell, K L, Hinman, R S, Metcalf, B R, Buchbinder, R, McConnell, J, McColl, G, Green, S, Crossley, K M (2005) Efficacy of physiotherapy management of knee joint osteoarthritis: a randomised, double blind, placebo controlled trial. Ann Rheum Dis, 64(6): 906–12.

Bennell, K, Duncan, M, Cowan, S (2006) Effect of patellar taping on vasti onset timing, knee kinematics, and kinetics in asymptomatic individuals with a delayed onset of vastus medialis oblique. Journal of Orthopaedic Research: official publication of the Orthopaedic Research Society, 1854–60.

Bewyer, D C, Bewyer, K J (2003) Rationale for treatment of hip abductor pain syndrome. Iowa Orthopaedic Journal, 23: 57–60.

Beynnon, B D, Vacek, P M, Murphy, D, Alosa, D, Paller, D (2005) First-time inversion ankle ligament trauma: the effects of sex, level of competition, and sport on the incidence of injury. American Journal of Sports Medicine, 33(10): 1485–91.

Biedert, R M, Warnke, K, Meyer, S (2003) Symphysis syndrome in athletes: surgical treatment for chronic lower abdominal, groin, and adductor pain in athletes. Clinical Journal of Sport Medicine, 13(5): 278–84.

Bohnsack, M, Halcour, A, Klages, P, Wilharm, A, Ostermeier, S, Ruhmann, O, Hurschler, C (2008) The influence of patellar bracing on patellar and knee load-distribution and kinematics: an experimental cadaver study. Knee Surgery, Sports Traumatology, Arthroscopy, 16(2): 135–41.

Brukner, P, Khan, K (2007) Clinical Sports Medicine. McGraw-Hill Australia, Sydney.

Bullock-Saxton, J E (1994) Local sensation changes and altered hip muscle function following severe ankle sprain. Physical Therapy, 74(1): 17–28; discussion 28–31.

Callaghan, M J, Selfe, J (2007) Has the incidence or prevalence of patellofemoral pain in the general population in the United Kingdom been properly evaluated? Physical Therapy in Sport, 8(1): 37–43.

Cleland, J A, Abbott, J H, Kidd, M O, Stockwell, S, Cheney, S, Gerrard, D F, Flynn, T W (2009) Manual physical therapy and exercise versus electrophysical agents and exercise in the management of plantar heel pain: a multicenter randomized clinical trial. Journal of Orthopaedic and Sports Physical Therapy, 39(8): 573–85.

Cook, J L, Khan, K M, Purdam, C R (2001) Conservative treatment of patellar tendinopathy. Physical Therapy in Sport, 2(2): 54–65.

Cowan, S M, Bennell, K L, Hodges, T W (2002) Therapeutic patellar taping changes the timing of vasti muscle activation in people with patellofemoral pain syndrome. Clinical Journal of Sport Medicine, 12(6): 339–47.

Cowan, S M, Hodges, P W, Crossley, K M, Bennell, K L (2006) Patellar taping does not change the amplitude of electromyographic activity of the vasti in a stair stepping task. British Journal of Sports Medicine, 30–4.

Crossley, K, Bennell, K, Green, S, Cowan, S, McConnell, J (2002) Physical therapy for patellofemoral pain — a randomized, double-blinded, placebo-controlled trial. American Journal of Sports Medicine, 30(6): 857–65.

Crossley, K, Marino, G, MacIlquham, M, Schache, A, Hinman, R (2009) The effect of patellar tape on patellar malalignment associated with patellofemoral osteoarthritis. Journal of Science and Medicine in Sport 12(suppl 1): S68.

Fagan, V, Delahunt, E (2008) Patellofemoral pain syndrome: a review on the associated neuromuscular deficits and current treatment options. British Journal of Sports Medicine, 42(10): 789–95.

Fairclough, J, Hayashi, K, Toumi, H, Lyons, K, Bydder, G, Phillips, N, Best, T M, Benjamin, M (2006) The functional anatomy of the iliotibial band during flexion and extension of the knee: implications for understanding iliotibial band syndrome. Journal of Anatomy, 208(3): 309–16.

Fong, D T, Man, C Y, Yung, P S, Cheung, S Y, Chan, K M (2008) Sport-related ankle injuries attending an accident and emergency department. Injury, 39(10): 1222–7.

Foucher, K C, Hurwitz, D E, Wimmer, M A, Foucher (2007) Preoperative gait adaptations persist one year after surgery in clinically well-functioning total hip replacement patients. Journal of Biomechanics, 40(15): 3432–7.

Franettovich, M, Chapman, A, Vicenzino, B (2008) Tape that increases medial longitudinal arch height also reduces leg muscle activity: a preliminary study. Medicine and Science in Sports and Exercise, 40(4): 593–600.

Gabrion, A, Jarde, O, Mertl, P, De Lestang, M (2003) Inferior dislocation of the proximal tibiofibular joint: a report on four cases. Acta Orthopaedica Belgica, 69(6): 522–7.

Grimaldi, A, Richardson, C, Durbridge, G, Donnelly, W, Darnell, R, Hides, J (2009) The association between degenerative hip joint pathology and size of the gluteus maximus and tensor fascia lata muscles. Manual Therapy, 14(6): 605–10.

Hardcastle, P, Nade, S (1985) The significance of the Trendelenburg test. Journal of Bone and Joint Surgery — British, 67(5): 741–6.

Harvey, G P, Woods, G W (1992) Antero-lateral dislocation of the proximal tibiofibular joint: case report and literature review. Todays OR Nurse, 14(3): 23–7.

Herrington, L, Al-Shammari, R A (2006) The effect of three degrees of elevation on swelling in acute inversion ankle sprains. Physical Therapy in Sport, 7(4): 175.

Herscovici, D, Jr, Fredrick, R W, Behrens, F (1992) Superior dislocation of the fibular head associated with a tibial shaft fracture. Journal Orthopaedic Trauma 6(1): 116–19.

Hinman, R S, Crossley, K M, McConnell, J, Bennell, K L (2003) Efficacy of knee tape in the management of osteoarthritis of the knee: blinded randomised controlled trial. British Medical Journal, 327(7407): 135.

Hubbard, T J, Hertel, J (2008) Anterior positional fault of the fibula after sub-acute lateral ankle sprains. Manual Therapy, 13(1): 63–7.

Hubbard, T J, Hicks-Little, C A (2008) Ankle ligament healing after an acute ankle sprain: an evidence-based approach. J Athl Train 43(5): 523–9.

Hudson, Z (2009) Iliotibial band tightness and patellofemoral pain syndrome: a case-control study. Manual Therapy, 14(2): 147–51.

Hudson, Z L, Darthuy, E (2006) Iliotibial band tightness and patellofemoral pain syndrome: a case-control study. Physical Therapy in Sport, 7(4): 173.

Ivins, D (2006) Acute ankle sprain: an update. American Family Physician 74(10): 1714–20.

Jamali, B, Walker, M, Hoke, B, Echternach, J (2004) Windlass taping technique for symptomatic relief of plantar fasciitis. Journal of Sports Rehabilitation, 13(3): 228–43.

Jennings, J, Davies, G J (2005) Treatment of cuboid syndrome secondary to lateral ankle sprains: a case series. The Journal of Orthopaedic and Sports Physical Therapy, (Alexandria, Va.) 35(7): 409–15.

Kavanagh, J (1999) Is there a positional fault at the inferior tibiofibular joint in patients with acute or chronic ankle sprains compared to normals? Manual Therapy, 4(1): 19–24.

Keet, J H L, Gray, J, Harley, Y, Lambert, M I (2007) The effect of medial patellar taping on pain, strength and neuromuscular recruitment in subjects with and without patellofemoral pain. Physiotherapy, 45–52.

Kilbreath, S L, Perkins, S, Crosbie, J, Mcconnell, J (2006) Gluteal taping improves hip extension during stance phase of walking following stroke. Australian Journal of Physiotherapy, 53–6.

Kingzett-Taylor, A, Tirman, P F, Feller, J, McGann, W, Prieto, V, Wischer, T, Cameron, J A, Cvitanic, O, Genant, H K (1999) Tendinosis and tears of gluteus medius and minimus muscles as a cause of hip pain: MR imaging findings. American Journal of Roentgenology, (Oct) 173: 1123–6.

Leinonen, V, Kankaanpaa, M, Airaksinen, O, Hanninen, O (2000) Back and hip extensor activities during trunk flexion/extension: effects of low back pain and rehabilitation. Archives of Physical Medicine and Rehabilitation, 81(1): 32–7.

Lievense, A, Bierma-Zeinstra, S, Schouten, B, Bohnen, A, Verhaar, J, Koes, B (2005) Prognosis of trochanteric pain in primary care. British Journal of General Practice, 55(512): 199–204.

Macgregor, K, Gerlach, S, Mellor, R, Hodges, P W (2005) Cutaneous stimulation from patella tape causes a differential increase in vasti muscle activity in people with patellofemoral pain. Journal of Orthopaedic Research, 23(2): 351–8.

Maitland, G D (2005) Peripheral Manipulation (4th edn). Butterworth–Heinemann, London.

Matzkin, E, Zachazewski, J E, Garrett, W E, Malone, T R (2007) Skeletal muscle: deformation, injury, repair and treatment considerations. In: D J Magee, J E Zachazewski, W S Quillen. Scientific Foundations and Principles of Practice in Musculoskeletal Rehabilitation. Saunders Elsevier, St Louis, 97–121.

Mazerolle, S M (2007) Cuboid syndrome in a college basketball player: a case report. Athletic Therapy Today, 12(6): 9–11.

McCarthy Persson, U, Fleming, H, Caulfield, B (2008) The effect of a vastus lateralis tape on muscle activity during stair climbing. Manual Therapy, 14(3) (June): 330–7.

McConnell, J (1986) The management of chondromalacia patellae: a long term solution. Australian Journal of Physiotherapy, 32: 215–23.

—— (2000) A novel approach to pain relief pre-therapeutic exercise. Journal of Science and Medicine in Sport, 3(3): 325–34.

—— (2002) Recalcitrant chronic low back and leg pain—a new theory and different approach to management. Manual Therapy, 7(4): 183–92.

McPoil, T G, Cornwall, M W, Vicenzino, B, Teyhen, D S, Molloy, J M, Christie, D S, Collins, N (2008) Effect of using truncated versus total foot length to calculate the arch height ratio. Foot, 18(4): 220–7.

Moen, M H, Tol, J L, Weir, A, Steunebrink, M, Winter, T C D (2009) Medial tibial stress syndrome: a critical review. Sports Medicine, 39(7): 523–46.

Moiler, K, Hall, T, Robinson, K (2006) The role of fibular tape in the prevention of ankle injury in basketball: a pilot study. Journal of Orthopaedic and Sports Physical Therapy, 36(9): 661–8.

Mooney, M, Maffey-Ward, L (1994) Cuboid plantar and dorsal subluxations: assessment and treatment. Journal of Orthopaedic and Sports Physical Therapy, 20(4): 220–6.

Mulligan, B (1999) Manual Therapy 'NAGS', 'SNAGS', 'MWMS' etc. Plane View Services, Wellington NZ.

Nicholas, S J, Tyler, T F (2002) Adductor muscle strains in sport. Sports Medicine, 32(5): 339–44.

O'Brien, T, Vicenzino, B (1998) A study of the effects of Mulligan's mobilization with movement treatment of lateral ankle pain using a case study design. Manual Therapy, 3(2): 78–84.

O'Leary, S, Carroll, M, Mellor, R, Scott, A, Vicenzino, B (2002) The effect of soft tissue deloading tape on thoracic spine pressure pain thresholds in asymptomatic subjects. Manual Therapy, 7(3): 150–3.

Olmsted, L C, Vela, L I, Denegar, C R, Hertel, J (2004) Prophylactic ankle taping and bracing: a numbers-needed-to-treat and cost-benefit analysis. Journal of Athletic Training, 39(1): 95–100.

O'Sullivan, K, Kennedy, N, O'Neill, E, Ni Mhainin, U (2008) The effect of low dye taping on rear foot motion and plantar pressure during the stance phase of gait. BMC Musculoskeletal Disorders, 9: article number 11.

Overington, M, Goddard, D, Hing, W (2006) A critical appraisal and literature critique on the effect of patellar taping: is patellar taping effective in the treatment of patellofemoral pain syndrome? (Provisional abstract). New Zealand Journal of Physiotherapy, 66–80.

Rarick, G, Bigley, G, Karst, R, Malina, R (1962) The measurable support of the ankle joint by conventional methods of taping. Journal of Bone Joint Surgery — American, 44(6): 1183–90.

Ross, H M, Jennifer, L L, Stacey, A M, Jason, C G (2007) Lower extremity mechanics of iliotibial band syndrome during an exhaustive run. Gait and Posture, 26(3): 407–13.

Segal, N A, Felson, D T, Torner, J C, Zhu, Y, Curtis, J R, Niu, J, Nevitt, M C (2007) Greater trochanteric pain syndrome: epidemiology and associated factors. Archives of Physical Medicine and Rehabilitation, 88(8): 988–92.

Strauss, E J, Campbell, K, Bosco, J A (2007) Analysis of the cross-sectional area of the adductor longus tendon: a descriptive anatomic study. American Journal of Sports Medicine, 35(6): 996–9.

Tobin, S, Robinson, G (2000) The effect of McConnell vastus lateralis inhibition taping technique on vastus lateralis and vastus medialis activity. Physiotherapy, 86(4): 174–83.

Vaes, P, De Boeck, F, Handelberg, F, Opdecam, P (1985) Comparative radiological study of the influence of ankle joint strapping and taping on ankle stability. Journal of Orthopaedic and Sports Physical Therapy, 7(3).

Vicenzino, B (2004) Foot orthotics in the treatment of lower limb conditions: a musculoskeletal physiotherapy perspective. Manual Therapy, 9(4): 185–96.

Vicenzino, B, et al (2003) Initial effects of elbow taping on pain-free grip strength and pressure pain threshold. Journal of Orthopaedic & Sports Physical Therapy, 33(7): 400–7.

Vicenzino, B, Franettovich, M, Mcpoil, T, Russell, T, Skardoon, G, Bartold, S J (2005) Initial effects of anti-pronation tape on the medial longitudinal arch during walking and running — commentary. British Journal of Sports Medicine, 39(12): 939–43.

Vicenzino, B, Griffiths, S, Griffiths, L, Hadley, A (2000) Effect of antipronation tape and temporary orthotic on vertical navicular height before and after exercise. Journal of Orthopaedic and Sports Physical Therapy, 30(6).

Walker, P, Kannangara, S, Bruce, W J M, Michael, D, Van der Wall, H (2007) Lateral hip pain: does imaging predict response to localized injection? Clinical Orthopaedics & Related Research, 457: 144–9.

Woodley, B L, Newsham-West, R J et al (2007) Chronic tendinopathy: effectiveness of eccentric exercise. British Journal of Sports Medicine, 41(4): 188–98; discussion 199.

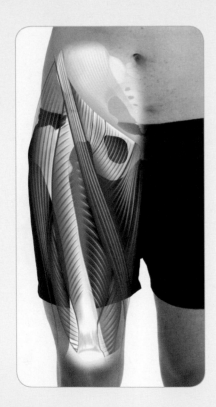
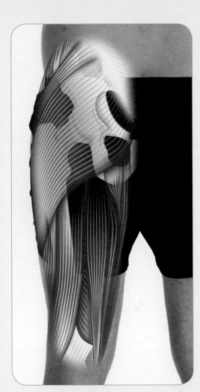

Cervical spine

Suboccipital and cervical extensor muscle deloading

Background and rationale

Thorough assessment of a patient with cervical spine pain may reveal pain-limited active range of motion (ROM) (Dall'Alba et al 2001) and pain at a spinal segmental level (Treleaven et al 1994). Similarly, some patients with neck conditions exhibit cervical muscle dysfunction (Falla 2004). Often clinical assessment will reveal, among other muscle dysfunction, tightness or overactivity of the cervical suboccipital muscles (Fernández-de-las-Peñas et al 2006). As an adjunct to usual therapy, this taping technique may be used to deload the suboccipital and cervical extensor muscles or to limit cervical active ROM to the pain-free range.

Evidence

O No research studies relating to this technique were identified.

Material

O Rigid tape 1 × 15 cm strip.
O Hypoallergenic underlay 1 × 15 cm may be used under the tape if preferred.

Patient position

O Patient is seated comfortably on a chair with pelvis in neutral position, the scapula set and the upper cervical spine in neutral position, with their eyes looking forward.
O Ensure patients with longer hair are able to lift and fix it above the posterior inferior hairline (to avoid entangling hair with tape).

Therapist position

O Therapist stands behind the patient.

68

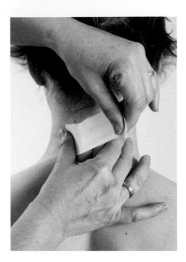

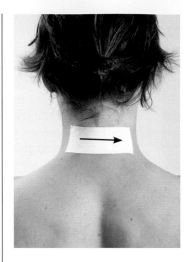

1 Apply a gentle deloading pressure to the left and right upper or lower cervical extensors using a 'lumbrical grip' with one hand.

2 The other hand applies the tape from the left to the right sides of the upper cervical extensors.

3 The tape can be applied to the suboccipital area if the aim of the technique is to deload the suboccipital muscles.

4 The tape can be applied at the level of any of the symptomatic zygapophyseal joints as described above.

Reassessment
○ Symptoms at rest.
○ Symptomatic active cervical ROM, provocative movement and symptoms.

Cervicothoracic fascial deloading

Background and rationale

Neck conditions with symptoms in the lower cervical spine may be associated with cervicothoracic (C-T) fascial pain. On clinical assessment the area may be tender to palpate around the cervicothoracic junction, the fascia may appear puffy and an increased cervicothoracic flexion may be apparent (Persson et al 2007). The increased activity of the surrounding muscles may add to the irritation of the fascia. In order to ascertain if the following technique will be of benefit to the patient, apply a deloading pressure around the cervicothoracic fascia using the thumb and index fingers held together in a diamond shape and ask the patient to perform the provocative cervical movement. If the range of motion has increased and/or the pain has decreased, then the following technique may be beneficial.

Evidence

- No research studies relating to this technique were identified.
- A randomised single blind placebo control study on asymptomatic subjects by O'Leary et al (2002) found that a 'box' deloading taping technique on the thoracic spine made no significant difference in pressure-pain thresholds (Level IV).
- Whereas Vicenzino et al (2003) found that in subjects with lateral epicondylalgia of the elbow a similar 'diamond' deloading taping technique significantly improved pain-free grip strength by 24% ($p = 0.028$) and improved pressure-pain threshold by 19% even though this was not statistically significant (Level IV).

Material

- Hypoallergenic underlay 4×10 cm strips.
- Rigid tape 8×10 cm strips.

Patient position

- Patient is seated comfortably on a chair with pelvis in neutral position, the scapula set and the upper cervical spine in neutral position, with their eyes looking forward.
- Ensure patients with longer hair are able to lift and fix it above the posterior hairline (to avoid entangling hair with tape).
- Alternative position: this technique may be performed with the patient in prone position with the face supported in a treatment bed face hole or on a rolled towel so the cervical spine is relaxed in neutral position. Arms of patient are resting by the patient's sides.

Therapist position

- Therapist stands behind the patient if patient is seated and beside the patient if patient is prone.

69

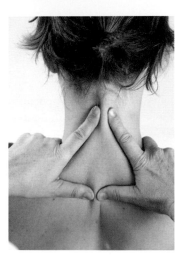

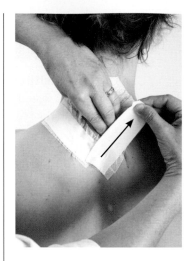

1 Apply 4 strips of hypoallergenic underlay in a diamond shape around the borders of the C-T fascia.
2 If patient consents it may be possible to draw lightly with a pen around the borders of the area to be taped (optional).

3 Apply a strip of tape over the hypoallergenic underlay on the inferior C-T fascia border, obliquely from inferior to superior with one hand, while the other hand simultaneously gathers and lifts the fascia upwards towards the centre of the diamond.
4 Repeat step 2 with a second strip of tape, applying it on the opposite inferior border of the C-T fascia from medial to lateral.

5 Apply a third strip of tape on the superior border of the fascia with one hand, while the other hand gathers and lifts the fascia towards the centre of the diamond.
6 Repeat step 4 with a fourth strip of tape, applying it on the opposite superior border of the C-T fascia, from lateral to medial.

69

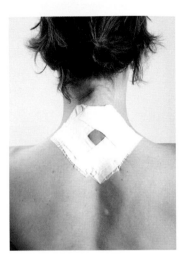

7 At the completion of the application of the four strips of tape the skin in the centre of the diamond should have a puckered appearance.

8 A second layer of tape overlapping by half the width of the previous tape may be applied over all four layers of tape to increase the deloading effect on the fascia.

Reassessment

○ Symptoms at rest.

○ Cervical, thoracic or shoulder active ROM, provocative movements and symptoms.

Thoracic spine

Thoracic spine box deloading technique

Background and rationale

Assessment of thoracic spine and cervical spine conditions may require manual palpation of the thoracic spinal segments and the surrounding soft tissues (Maitland 2005). Patients with ongoing pain in the thoracic area may become hyperalgesic and not be able to tolerate palpation of the area. Box deloading tape technique may be used as an adjunct to other usual treatment to unload the tender soft tissues on the thoracic spine (McConnell 2000; O'Leary et al 2002).

Evidence

- No research studies relating to this technique were identified.
- A randomised single blind placebo control study on asymptomatic subjects by O'Leary et al (2002) found that a 'box' deloading taping technique on the thoracic spine made no significant difference in pressure-pain thresholds (Level IV)
- Whereas Vicenzino et al (2003) found that in subjects with lateral epicondylalgia of the elbow a similar 'diamond' deloading taping technique significantly improved pain-free grip strength by 24% ($p = 0.028$) and improved pressure-pain threshold by 19% even though this was not statistically significant (Level IV).

Material

- Hypoallergenic underlay 4 × 10 cm strips.
- Rigid tape 8 × 10 cm strips.

Patient position

- Patient lies prone with the face supported in a treatment bed face hole or on a rolled towel so the cervical spine is relaxed in neutral position.
- Alternatively this can be performed with the patient seated comfortably on a chair with pelvis in neutral position, the scapula set and the upper cervical spine in neutral position, with their eyes looking forward.
- Ensure patients with longer hair are able to lift and fix it above the posterior hairline (to avoid entangling hair with tape).

Therapist position

- Therapist stands beside or behind the patient.

70

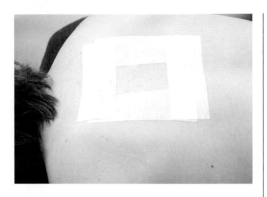

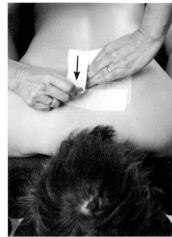

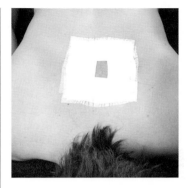

1   Identify the areas of the thoracic spine that are sensitive, hyperalgesic or painful.
2   If patient consents it may be possible to draw lightly with a pen around the borders of the area to be taped.
3   Apply 4 strips of hypoallergenic underlay in a square shape around the borders of the area to be taped.
4   Apply a strip of tape over the hypoallergenic underlay on the inferior border of the 'square' and/or 'box' in a horizontal direction from left to right, or the reverse, with one hand while the other hand simultaneously gathers and lifts the superficial tissues upwards towards the centre of the square (towards the spinous processes).

5   Apply a second strip of tape on the left or right border of the square with one hand, from inferior to superior direction, while the other hand gathers and lifts the fascia towards the centre of the square.
6   Repeat step 5 with a third strip of tape, applying it on the opposite border of the square.
7   Repeat step 4 with a fourth strip of tape, applying it on the superior border of the square.

8   At the completion of the application of the four strips of tape the skin in the centre of the 'box' should have a puckered appearance.
9   A second layer of tape overlapping by half the width of the previous tape may be applied over all four layers of tape to increase the deloading effect on the superficial thoracic spine tissues.

Reassessment
○   Symptoms at rest.
○   Tenderness on palpation of thoracic spinous process and surrounding soft tissue.
○   Cervical, thoracic or shoulder active ROM, provocative movements and symptoms.

70

Erector spinae facilitation

Background and rationale

In certain spinal conditions there may be changes in the motor activity of the erector spinae muscles. It has been shown for instance that erector spinae thoracic muscle segments have greater fatiguability than the lumbar spine segments in patients with low back pain (Sung et al 2009). It has also been shown that in patients with scoliosis there is higher paraspinal muscle bulk on the concave side of the scoliosis (Zoabli et al 2007) and a side to side difference in the activation of the erector spinae muscles (Avikainen et al 1999). It is thus important that the management of patients with low back pain or with the presence of scoliosis does address any observed differences in erector spinae muscle activation.

This simple technique uses a single strip of tape placed along a segment of the erector spinae. It is anticipated that the tape will provide the patient with increased awareness of the area of erector spinae that requires increased motor activity for postural correction or a required exercise, movement and task. Taping is done only as an adjunct to other therapeutic management of the spine.

Evidence

O No research studies relating to this technique were identified.

Material

O Hypoallergenic underlay 2 × 15–20 cm strips.
O Alternatively, tape 2 × 15–20 cm strips.

Patient position

O Patient is seated, feet well supported, pelvis and lumbar spine in neutral position and scapula set in neutral, cervical spine in neutral with eyes looking straight ahead.
O Alternatively, patient is in a standing position, feet comfortably apart, pelvis and lumbar spine in neutral position, scapulae set in neutral, cervical spine in neutral, with eyes looking straight ahead.

Therapist position

O Standing behind the patient.

71

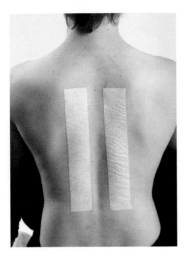

1 Apply one or two longitudinal strips of hypoallergenic underlay along the length of the section of the erector spinae that requires increased motor activity (thoracic spine or lumbar spine), applying gently and lightly.

2 Alternatively, rigid strapping tape may be applied directly to the skin in a similar fashion, ensuring light application on the skin.

Reassessment

○ Provocative movement and symptoms.
○ Patient awareness and activation of erector spinae muscle during postural correction or a particular exercise.

71

Lumbar spine

Lumbar spine support

Background and rationale

Clinical assessment of lumbar spine may reveal patients are experiencing pain at rest and during active ROM. Taping may be an adjunct to usual treatment (Mulligan 1999; McConnell 2002; Brukner & Khan 2007). This technique may be applied with only one layer of tape in the shape of an X around the lumbar spine, or with multiple layers of tape in the shape of an X, reinforced with tape in the shape of a square around the X. How much tape is used will depend on the purpose the taping technique is intended for. An increased amount of tape will provide more restriction to certain lumbar spine movements and a decreased amount of tape will act mainly to increase patient awareness and proprioception of the area where specific exercise needs to be addressed, such as specific multifidus muscle activation (Hides & Richardson 2003).

Evidence

○ No research studies that investigated the effects of lumbar spine taping were identified.

Material

○ Hypoallergenic underlay 4 × 10–15cm strips.
○ Rigid tape 10 × 10–15 cm strips.

Patient position

○ Patient standing with feet slightly apart, pelvis in neutral position, scapulae in neutral position and head looking straight ahead.
○ Alternatively, if the patient is unable to stand for a few minutes due to pain, the technique can be performed with the patient in a prone position.

Therapist position

○ Standing behind the patient or beside the patient.

72

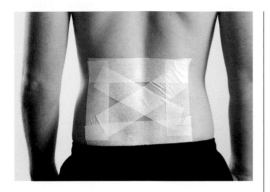 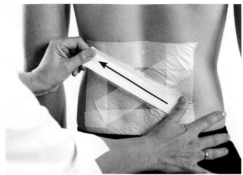 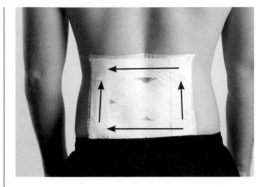

1 Apply hypoallergenic underlay in the shape of an X over the lumbar spine, the centre of the X being over the symptomatic lumbar level.
2 Apply hypoallergenic underlay in the shape of a square around the X, joining the four edges of the cross.

3 Apply tape over the X of the hypoallergenic underlay, from inferior to superior, ensuring the tape is taut as it is placed on the patient.

4 If the aim is to provide increased support to the lumbar spine, a second and a third layer of tape in the shape of a cross may be applied over the first layer of tape.
5 Apply tape over the square of the hypoallergenic underlay as a lock-off.

Reassessment
○ Symptoms at rest.
○ Lumbar spine active ROM, functional symptomatic tasks and symptoms.

72

Thoracolumbar fascial deloading

Background and rationale

The posterior thoracolumbar fascia is interrelated with gluteus maximus, latissimus dorsi and the erector spinae muscles (Vleeming et al 1995). Based on the activity of the muscles interrelated with the thoracolumbar fascia the resultant tightness of the fascia may contribute to lumbar spine active ROM limitation in patients experiencing low back symptoms. Tape may be used as a fascial deloading technique to unload the thoracolumbar fascia by being applied around the fascia in a 'diamond' shape.

Evidence

- No research studies relating to this technique were identified.
- A randomised single blind placebo control study on asymptomatic subjects by O'Leary et al (2002) found that a 'box' deloading taping technique on the thoracic spine made no significant difference in pressure-pain thresholds (Level IV).
- Whereas Vicenzino et al (2003) found that in subjects with lateral epicondylalgia of the elbow a similar 'diamond' deloading taping technique significantly improved pain-free grip strength by 24% ($p = 0.28$) and improved pressure-pain threshold by 19% even though this was not statistically significant (Level IV).

Material

- Hypoallergenic underlay 4×10 cm strips.
- Rigid tape 8×10 cm strips.

Patient position

- Patient is prone with pelvis in neutral position.

Therapist position

- Therapist stands beside the patient.

73

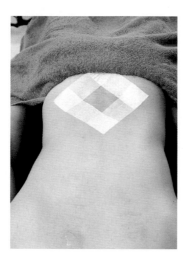 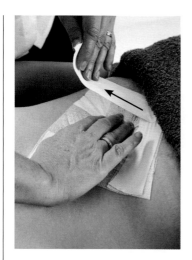 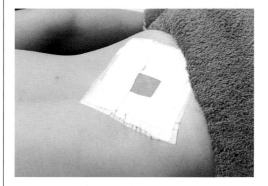

1 Apply 4 strips of hypoallergenic underlay in a diamond shape around the borders of the thoracolumbar fascia.

2 Apply a strip of tape over the hypoallergenic underlay on the inferior thoracolumbar fascia border, obliquely from inferior to superior with one hand, while the other hand simultaneously gathers and lifts the fascia upwards towards the centre of the diamond.

3 Repeat step 2 with a second strip of tape, applying it on the opposite inferior border of the thoracolumbar fascia.

4 Apply a third strip of tape on the superior border of the fascia with one hand, while the other hand gathers and lifts the fascia towards the centre of the diamond.

5 Repeat step 4 with a fourth strip of tape, applying it on the opposite superior border of the thoracolumbar fascia.

6 At the completion of the application of the four strips of tape the skin in the centre of the diamond should have a puckered appearance.

7 A second layer of tape overlapping by half the width of the previous tape may be applied over all four layers of tape to increase the deloading effect on the fascia.

Reassessment

○ Symptoms at rest.
○ Thoracic and lumbar spine active range of motion, provocative movements and symptoms.

73

Lumbar spine zygapophyseal (facet) joint deloading

Background and rationale

Assessment of patients with lumbar spine conditions may involve manual palpation and accessory joint glides of the spinal segments (Maitland 2005). Patients with severe pain and tenderness on a particular spinal segment may not tolerate palpation well. Box deloading tape technique (McConnell 2000; O'Leary et al 2002) may be used as an adjunct to usual treatment to unload the tender soft tissues on the lumbar spine zygapophyseal joint.

Evidence

- No research studies relating to this technique were identified.
- Some studies that related to the principle of deloading or muscle inhibition support the general principle of reducing load on injured tissues with tape in other body regions, such as the thoracic spine (O' Leary et al 2002) and lateral epicondylalgia of the elbow (Vicenzino et al 2003). The outcomes of these studies are described in Chapter 2.

Material

- Hypoallergenic underlay 4 × 5 cm strips.
- Rigid tape 8 × 5 cm strips.

Patient position

- Patient lies prone with pelvis in comfortable pain-free position. A pillow under the abdomen may further assist in relieving low back pain.

Therapist position

- Therapist stands beside the patient.

74

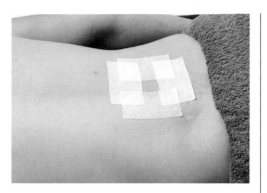

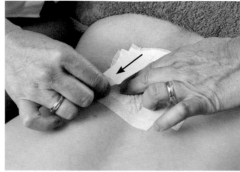

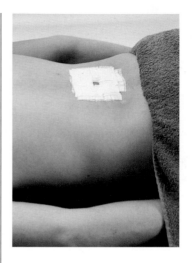

1   Identify the symptomatic side and level of the lumbar spine zygapophyseal joint.
2   If the patient consents it may be possible to draw with a pen around the borders of the area to be taped.
3   Apply four strips of hypoallergenic underlay in a square shape, ensuring the zygapophyseal joint is in the centre of the square.
4   Apply a strip of tape over the hypo-allergenic underlay on the inferior border of the 'square' or 'box' in a horizontal direction from left to right, or the reverse, with one hand while the other hand simultaneously gathers and lifts the superficial tissues up-wards towards the centre of the square (towards the zygapophyseal joint).

5   Apply a second strip of tape on the left or right border of the square with one hand, from inferior to superior direction, while the other hand gathers and lifts the fascia towards the centre of the square.
6   Repeat step 5 with a third strip of tape, applying it on the opposite border of the square.
7   Repeat step 4 with a fourth strip of tape, applying it on the superior border of the square.

8   At the completion of the application of the four strips of tape the skin in the centre of the square should have a puckered appearance.
9   A second layer of tape overlapping by half the width of the previous tape may be applied over all four layers of tape to increase the deloading effect on the zygapophyseal joint.

Reassessment
○ Patient's symptoms at rest.
○ Lumbar spine active range of motion, provocative movements and symptoms experienced during movement.

74

Pelvis and sacroiliac joint

Pelvis neutral position

Background and rationale

Re-education for posture may be undertaken for different cervical, thoracic and lumbar spine, pelvis, hip, knee and shoulder conditions. When postural re-education is undertaken either in sitting or in standing positions attaining the lumbar spine and pelvis neutral position is one of the initial strategies frequently taught by therapists (Lam et al 1999; Claus et al 2009). When a patient is having difficulty attaining neutral pelvis position with usual instructions or cueing, tape can be used as an adjunct to assist in increasing awareness of the required position.

Evidence

○ No research studies relating to this taping technique were identified.

Material

○ Hypoallergenic underlay 2 × 55–60 cm strips and 1 × 35–40 cm strip.
○ Tape 2 × 55–60 cm strips and 1 × 35–40 cm strip.

Patient position

○ Patient is standing with feet slightly apart and positioned with pelvis in neutral.

Therapist position

○ Standing behind the patient.

75

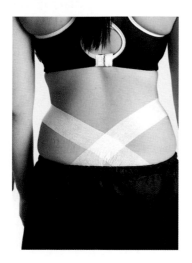
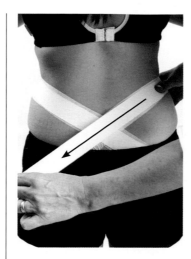
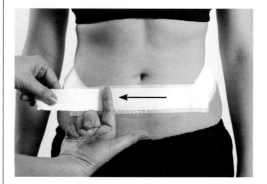

1 Apply two strips of hypoallergenic underlay from each anterior superior iliac spine (ASIS), directing the tape diagonally and posteriorly crossing each sacroiliac joint (SIJ), finishing the tape on the contralateral buttock. Ensure the two strips of hypoallergenic underlay cross each other over the sacrum.

2 Apply a strip of tape over the hypoallergenic underlay, starting at the ASIS, tensioning the tape and applying in the same direction as the hypoallergenic underlay.

3 Repeat step 2 for the contra lateral.

4 Apply a strip of hypoallergenic underlay tape anteriorly in a horizontal direction from one ASIS to the other.

5 Apply a strip of tape over the hypoallergenic underlay on one ASIS, tension it and finish it on the other ASIS, ensuring the patient has maintained the pelvis neutral position during the application of the technique.

Reassessment

○ Patient's symptoms at rest.
○ Lumbar spine active ROM, provocative movements and symptoms experienced during movement.
○ Patient's ability to position pelvis in neutral during sitting and standing positions.

75

Sacroiliac joint support

Background and rationale

Sacroiliac joint (SIJ) pain may be associated with SIJ hypo-mobility or hyper-mobility. A thorough assessment of the SIJ and lumbar spine is needed to establish the relationship of low back pain and SIJ mobility status (Foley & Buschbacher 2006). As an adjunct to usual treatment, SIJ stability belts (Lee 2004; Foley & Buschbacher 2006) and abdominal muscle activation (Richardson et al 2002) are used by therapists to provide passive and dynamic support to hyper-mobile SIJs. Taping can be used as an adjunct to the usual treatment (Lee 2004) and it may be useful also in cases where SIJ stability belts are unavailable for providing temporary support to a hyper-mobile SIJ.

Evidence

○ No research studies relating to this technique were identified.

Material

○ Hypoallergenic underlay 2 × 55–60 cm strips.
○ Tape 2 × 55–60 cm strips.

Patient position

○ Patient is standing with feet slightly apart and positioned with pelvis in neutral.

Therapist position

○ The therapist stands behind the patient to apply the hypoallergenic underlay and moves to the side of the patient while applying the tape.

76

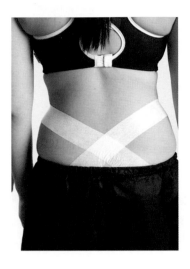 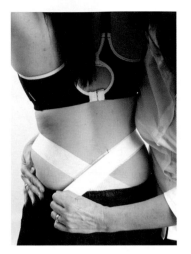 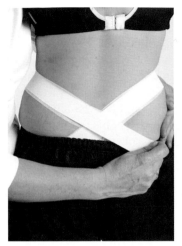 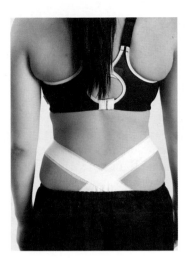

1 Apply two strips of hypoallergenic underlay from each anterior superior iliac spine (ASIS), directing the tape diagonally and posteriorly crossing the ipsilateral and the contralateral sacroiliac joints (SIJ), finishing the tape on the contralateral buttock.

2 Ensure the two strips of hypoallergenic underlay cross each other over the sacrum.

3 Apply a strip of tape over the hypoallergenic underlay, starting at the ASIS.

4 Move and stand to the side of the patient (same side as the tape being applied), and with one hand tension the tape while with the other hand you approximate the pelvis and two SIJs together.

5 Apply the tensioned tape over the hypoallergenic underlay in a posterior diagonal direction, finishing on the contralateral buttock.

6 Repeat with the second tape on the other SIJ, while maintaining the approximating force of the two SIJs and pelvis.

Reassessment
○ Patient's symptoms at rest.
○ Lumbar spine active ROM, provocative movements and symptoms experienced during movement.

76

Sacroiliac joint innominate anterior and posterior glide

Background and rationale

The usual assessment of sacroiliac joint (SIJ) related conditions includes evaluation of SIJ and sacrum mobility (Maitland 2005). The treatment approach may include an antero-posterior or a postero-anterior accessory glide of the innominate on the sacrum which may result in patient symptom relief (Lee 2004). Tape can be used as an adjunct to usual management and post mobilisation of the innominate to provide support to the SIJ. This taping technique can be done only on the affected side as a unilateral technique. If indicated, taping can be performed on the unaffected side and applying only the approximating force to the SIJs and pelvis as in the previous technique (technique 76).

Evidence

○ No research studies relating to this technique were identified.

Material

○ Hypoallergenic underlay $1 \times 55-60$ cm strips.
○ Tape $1 \times 55-60$ cm strips.

Patient position

○ Patient is standing with feet slightly apart and positioned with pelvis in neutral.

Therapist position

○ Standing to the side of the patient that is to be taped.

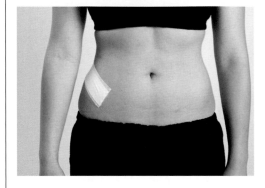

For antero-posterior innominate rotation glide

1 Apply a strip of hypoallergenic underlay from the anterior superior iliac spine (ASIS) of the affected side, directing the tape diagonally and posteriorly crossing the ipsilateral and the contralateral sacroiliac joints (SIJ), finishing the tape on the contralateral buttock.

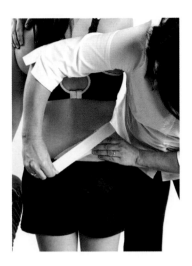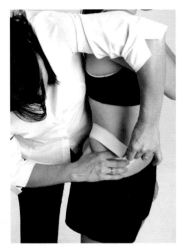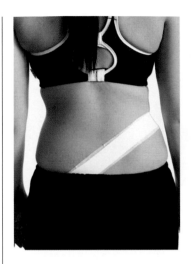

For antero-posterior innominate rotation glide

2 Apply a strip of tape over the hypoallergenic underlay, starting at the ASIS.

3 With one hand, tension the tape while the other hand applies a posterior accessory rotation glide of the innominate.

4 Apply the tensioned tape over the hypoallergenic underlay in a posterior diagonal direction, finishing on the contralateral buttock.

For postero-anterior innominate rotation glide

5 Apply a strip of tape over the hypoallergenic underlay, starting at the contralateral buttock.

6 With one hand, tension the tape while the other hand applies an anterior accessory rotation glide of the innominate.

7 Apply the tensioned tape over the hypoallergenic underlay in an anterior diagonal direction, finishing on the ipsilateral ASIS.

8 If it is indicated, the other SIJ may be taped without applying a rotation accessory glide as described in the technique above.

77

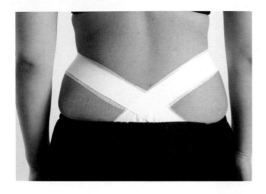

Reassessment

○ Patient's symptoms at rest.
○ Lumbar spine active ROM, provocative
  movements and symptoms experienced
  during movement.

REFERENCES

Avikainen, V J, Rezasoltani, A, Kauhanen, H A (1999) Asymmetry of paraspinal EMG-time characteristics in idiopathic scoliosis. Journal of Spinal Disorders, 12(1): 61–67.

Brukner, P, Khan, K (2007) Clinical Sports Medicine (3rd edn). McGraw-Hill Australia, Sydney.

Claus, A P, Hides, J A, Moseley, G L, Hodges, P W (2009) Is 'ideal' sitting posture real? Measurement of spinal curves in four sitting postures. Manual Therapy, 14(4): 404–8.

Dall'Alba, P T, Sterling, M M, Treleaven, J M, Edwards, S L, Jull, G A (2001) Cervical range of motion discriminates between asymptomatic persons and those with whiplash. Spine, 26(19): 2090–4.

Falla, D (2004) Unravelling the complexity of muscle impairment in chronic neck pain. Manual Therapy, 9(3): 125–33.

Fernández-de-las-Peñas, C, Alonso-Blanco, C, Luz Cuadrado, M, Pareja, J A (2006) Myofascial trigger points in the suboccipital muscles in episodic tension-type headache. Manual Therapy, 11(3): 225–30.

Foley, B S, Buschbacher, R M (2006) Sacroiliac joint pain: anatomy, biomechanics, diagnosis, and treatment. American Journal of Physical Medicine & Rehabilitation, 85(12): 997–1006.

Hides, J A, Richardson, C A (2003) Segmental stabilization training in lumbo-pelvic pain disorders. New Zealand Journal of Sports Medicine, 31(1): 10–18.

Lam, S S, Jull, G, Treleaven, J (1999) Lumbar spine kinesthesia in patients with low back pain. Journal of Orthopaedic & Sports Physical Therapy, 29(5): 294–9.

Lee, D (2004) The pelvic girdle: an approach to the examination and treatment of the lumbopelvic-hip region. Churchill Livingstone, Edinburgh.

Maitland, G D (2005) Spinal manipulation. Butterworth–Heinemann, London.

McConnell, J (2000) A novel approach to pain relief pre-therapeutic exercise. Journal of Science and Medicine in Sport, 3(3): 325–34.

McConnell, J (2002) Recalcitrant chronic low back and leg pain — a new theory and different approach to management. Manual Therapy, 7(4): 183–92.

Mulligan, B (1999) Manual Therapy 'NAGs', 'SNAGs', 'MWMs' etc. Plane View Services, Wellington.

O' Leary, S, Carroll, M, Mellor, R, Scott, A, Vicenzino, B (2002) The effect of soft tissue deloading tape on thoracic spine pressure-pain thresholds in asymptomatic subjects. Manual Therapy, 7(3): 150–3.

Persson, P R, Hirschfeld, H et al (2007) Associated sagittal spinal movements in performance of head pro- and retraction in healthy women: a kinematic analysis. Manual Therapy, 12(2): 119–25.

Richardson, C A, Snijders, C J, Hides, J A, Damen, L, Pas, M S, Storm, J (2002) The relation between the transversus abdominis muscles, sacroiliac joint mechanics, and low back pain. Spine, 27(4): 399–405.

Sung, P S, Lammers, A R, Danial, P (2009) Different parts of erector spinae muscle fatiguability in subjects with and without low back pain. The Spine Journal, 9(2): 115–20.

Treleaven, J, Jull, G, Atkinson, L (1994) Cervical musculoskeletal dysfunction in post-concussional headache. Cephalalgia, 14(4): 273–9.

Vicenzino, B, Brooksbank, J, Minto, J, Offord, S, Paungmali, A (2003) Initial effects of elbow taping on pain-free grip strength and pressure. Journal of Orthopaedic & Sports Physical Therapy, 33(7): 400–7.

Vleeming, A, Pool-Goudzwaard, A L, Stoeckart, R, van Wingerden, J P, Snijders, C J (1995) The posterior layer of the thoracolumbar fascia: its function in load transfer from spine to legs. Spine, 20(7): 753–8.

Zoabli, G, Mathieu, P A, Aubin, C-É (2007) Back muscles biometry in adolescent idiopathic scoliosis. The Spine Journal, 7(3): 338–44.

CHAPTER 7
Soft casting techniques

Soft cast tape is useful in providing semi-rigid immobilisation in certain musculoskeletal conditions. Soft cast is made from knitted fibreglass material which contains a polyurethane resin with a water soluble lubricant (Schuren 1994). As described by Jan Schuren (1994), exposure of the resin 'to ambient temperature or water initiates a chemical reaction which causes the resin to set'. Once set the cast remains soft while still retaining its shape and resilience. Some of the therapeutic applications of soft cast tape include, but are not limited to, using it after removal of a rigid cast (Neugebauer et al 1995) to allow more movement while still providing immobilisation of the injured area, as a brace or splint (Khan et al 2007) or in place of taping (Walters et al 2008). Soft cast tape can be particularly useful in patients who have known sensitivity or develop sensitivity to the rigid adhesive tape. A number of taping techniques can be adapted and applied using soft cast tape, particularly in musculoskeletal conditions of the wrist, hand, ankle and foot regions.

Research in the use of soft cast is limited. A recent randomised trial compared soft and rigid casts in the management of buckle fractures of the distal radius in 117 children (Khan et al 2007). Both groups fully recovered after 3 weeks of casting. The families and the children reported satisfaction with the use of soft cast, which allowed the parents to remove it at home and reduced the need for a follow-up hospital appointment. The authors concluded that buckle fractures of the wrist can be treated safely with soft cast.

Another within-subjects cohort study recently investigated changes in plantar pressures with low dye soft cast application during gait (Walters et al 2008). The study included 32 subjects with greater than 10 mm navicular drop used as a measure of foot pronation. The authors concluded that the use of soft cast had an effect on plantar pressures and could be considered as an alternative management approach to controlling foot pronation (Walters et al 2008).

In some contact sports soft cast is considered safe for players to wear on the field. It is advisable that therapists check with the rules and regulations of particular sports to ensure soft cast use is allowable during play.

As described in Chapter 3, informed consent and precautionary warning processes described for the use of taping need to be also adhered to when intending to use soft cast applications.

PRECAUTIONS IN SOFT CASTING

Contact of soft cast material with the skin or eyes just before it sets may cause irritation and care must thus be taken by both the therapist and the patient to avoid touching the material. The soft cast tape is removed from its sealed package one roll at a time. It is recommended that gloves are worn by the therapist when handling the soft cast and that the patient is protected with thin layered tubular bandage material, such as a stockinet worn over the body region to be treated. If the therapist's or patient's skin comes into contact with the soft cast resin, it is advisable to remove the resin immediately using a light isopropyl alcohol swab (Schuren 1994). Once the soft cast material has been exposed to the atmosphere or water, the therapist should work quickly as it will begin to set within minutes. Soft cast is safe for skin contact when set.

Soft cast should not be used in cases where the patient has:
- known skin allergy or sensitivity to fibreglass material
- open wounds

Precaution should be used when using soft cast in cases where the patient has:
- skin infections/conditions; for example, dermatitis, eczema
- diabetes
- peripheral vascular disease
- peripheral neuropathies
- circulatory conditions — bleeding or clotting disorders
- prolonged use of steroid or anticoagulant medication
- fragile or sensitive skin which is prone to tears and bruising.

PATIENT WARNING AND CONSENT

Standard practice of gaining informed consent as described in Chapter 3 must be followed prior to the application of soft cast tape. After application, it is essential the therapist ensures the cast is comfortable at rest and during movement, and also checks circulation has not been impaired. A similar warning to that used for taping applies, ensuring the patient understands and is aware of when and how to remove the cast. This can be modified from the following sample warning:

You may leave the cast on for ..... days/weeks. The cast can become wet if you wish to swim or shower with it on. However, you must ensure the cast is adequately dry prior to being covered. If at any time you are experiencing
- additional discomfort
- increase in any of your symptoms
- feelings of pins and needles or numbness at the site of the cast or around the area of the cast
- feelings of skin itchiness or irritability under the cast
- skin colour changes around the cast such as pallor, redness or blueness, and/or
- increased swelling around the cast

you must remove the cast immediately. The cast can be removed by using a pair of scissors to cut through the cast from one end to another. If you have any concerns regarding the application and removal of this cast please feel free to contact me.

Do you understand this warning? Do you have any questions?

PREPARATION AND MATERIAL FOR SOFT CAST APPLICATION

The material required for the soft casting should be prepared in advance and placed within easy reach of the treatment area. The patient should be placed in a comfortable position to enable the required casting technique to be applied and the relevant limb to be treated should be clean and dry. Shaving of bodily hair is not necessary for soft casting. The main materials required for soft casting are:

- soft cast tape rolls; for example, 5 cm width for fingers and hand, 7.5 cm for ankle and foot
- thin stockinet to be worn under the cast by the patient (5 cm and 2 cm width)
- high density adhesive foam to be used under soft cast to protect bony prominences
- plastic disposable gloves
- room temperature water in a small deep bowl
- blunt nose scissors for trimming and/or removing
- one short shoelace if it is to be a reusable splint.

The following three soft casting techniques are a small sample of the many techniques therapists may be able to adapt and use as therapeutic applications.

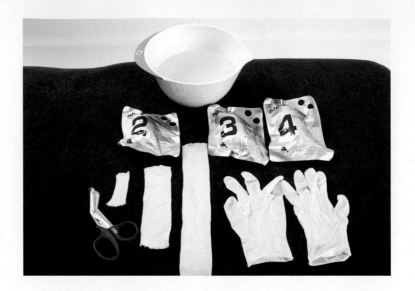

Thumb soft cast splint

Background and rationale

Carpometacarpal (CMC) joint osteoarthritis and thumb ulnar or radial collateral ligament injuries of the metacarpophalangeal (MCP) joint may be associated with painful functional activities. Usual management may incorporate immobilisation of the CMC or the MCP joints for a period of time. In Chapter 4 several variations of taping were described to address immobilisation of these joints. However, it may be necessary to use soft cast instead of tape in cases where:

○ the patient has developed an allergic reaction to tape
○ the patient is returning to sport and requires increased support
○ the patient is awaiting a splint to be delivered and repeated tape use is not an option.

Evidence

○ No research studies relating to the effects of soft cast on the management of thumb conditions were identified.

Material

○ Soft cast material 2.5 cm, ensuring packet is sealed.
○ Cotton stockinet, 7 × 2.5 cm and 7 × 5 cm to be worn under soft cast.
○ Soft dense foam for padding if necessary.
○ Plastic gloves.
○ Room temperature water in a small bowl.
○ Blunt nose scissors for trimming and/or removing.
○ One short shoelace if soft cast is to be reusable.

Patient position

○ Patient seated with elbow flexed, resting on a table, hand and thumb held in the functional position.

Therapist position

○ Therapist is seated or standing in front of the patient.

78

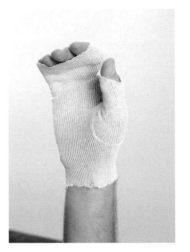
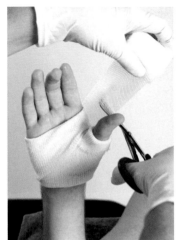
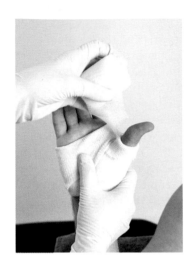
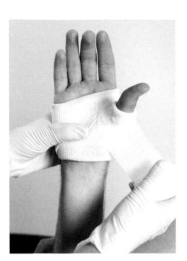

1   Measure and cut stockinet:
   1.1 from the fingers to the carpus using 5 cm width stockinet
   1.2 the length of the thumb using the 2.5 cm width stockinet.
2   Apply hand and thumb stockinet on patient's hand.
3   Put plastic gloves on.
4   Open soft cast packet and take soft cast out.
5   Start by rolling the soft cast tape like a bandage, applying it to the wrist, ensuring the soft cast is taut without being pulled hard, moving up to the thumb in a half figure 8, across the palm to below the metacarpal heads.
6   Overlap each previous layer by half the width of the new layer.
7   You may use scissors to cut a slit in the soft cast in order to spread it around the web space.
8   Fold the edges of the stockinet at the wrist and at the distal phalanx back onto the soft cast and apply a layer of soft cast over the stockinet to set it in place.
9   When finished applying the technique, cut off the remaining unused soft cast.

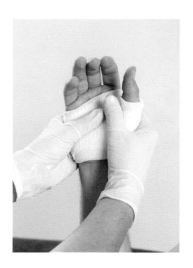 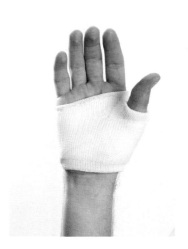 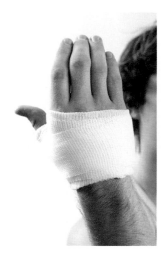 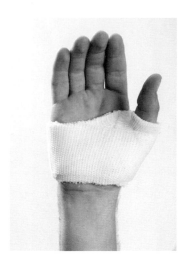

10 Wet hands in room temperature water and with the wet hands mould soft cast onto hand, making sure it is a firm fit (ensure you do not press too hard on the soft cast material so that you form impressions on the cast, as this may cause potential pressure areas).

11 Trim soft cast splint to the level of the CMC joint line, so wrist flexion and extension is not impaired.

12 Trim soft cast splint around the thumb proximal phalanx to ensure the interphalangeal (IP) joint flexion and extension of the thumb is not impaired.

13 Wait 5–10 minutes until the soft cast sets.

14 Soft cast splint may be left on for a few days or several weeks depending on the clinical indication. It may get wet without being damaged.

78

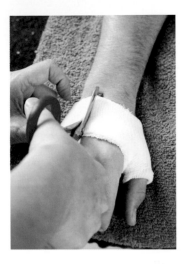

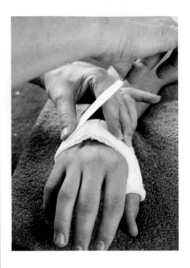

15 If soft cast is to be used as a reusable splint it may be cut off with blunt nose scissors using a vertical slit on the dorsal aspect to remove it.

16 Trim any rough edges of the soft cast splint to suit the patient's comfort, ensuring it allows the patient to grip and to oppose fingers.

17 Puncture holes in the dorsal side and use a shoelace to tie the soft cast splint edges together when worn.

Follow-up
○ Splint may be left on for several days.
○ Splint may be removed with blunt nose scissors by cutting it on the dorsal side.

Reassessment
○ Patient circulation of thumb, fingers and hand.
○ Patient comfort and symptoms at rest.
○ Thumb opposition and grip strength.
○ Thumb IP joint and wrist flexion and extension ROM should not be hindered.

Ankle soft cast

Background and rationale

Taping, bracing or splinting may be an adjunct to usual management of ankle injuries such as lateral ankle and high ankle sprains (Edwards & DeLee 1984; Simpson et al 1999; Kerkhoffs et al 2002) or after removal of rigid cast for ankle fracture immobilisation. Another option for ankle splinting is soft cast and it may be used when:

- tape has caused an allergic skin reaction
- repeated tape use is not an option
- where a brace is not available and a player is returning back to sport and requires added support
- while awaiting the delivery of a brace
- it is preferred by the player.

Evidence

- No research studies relating to the effects of soft cast on the management of ankle conditions were identified.

Material

- Soft cast material 5 or 7.5 cm (2 or 3 inch) width.
- Cotton 7.5 cm (3 inch) stockinet to be worn under soft cast (as scotch-cast material may cause skin irritability).
- Soft dense foam for padding if necessary.
- Plastic gloves.
- Room temperature water in a small bowl.
- Blunt nose scissors for trimming and/or removing.
- One small shoelace if it is to be a reusable splint.

Patient position

- Patient seated or supine on a treatment bed, with the foot over the edge of the bed.

Therapist position

- Standing or seated in front of the foot of the patient. Ensure all materials are within easy reach.

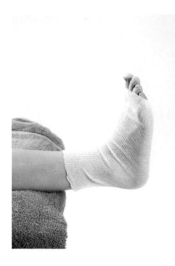 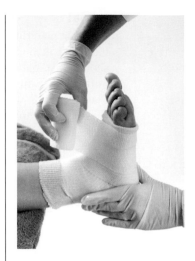 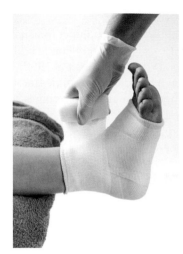

1 Measure, cut and apply 7.5 cm stockinet to the ankle and foot (up to 8–10 cm above the malleoli).
2 Use soft dense foam around bony prominences such as the malleoli and over the tendo-Achilles.
3 Put plastic gloves on.

4 Open 5 cm soft cast tape and roll it out like a bandage, applying from the base of the toes at the foot, distal to proximal in figure of 8s, around foot while ensuring there is no tension.
5 Apply soft cast material up to approximately 5–8 cm above the malleoli.
6 Overlap each previous layer by half the width of the new layer.
7 When soft cast application is finished, wet hands in cold water and start moulding the splint, pressing around all the bony prominences firmly.
8 Trim soft cast splint to the level of the metatarsophalangeal (MTP) joints, so toe flexion and extension is not impaired.
9 Trim soft cast splint around the ankle.
10 Wait 5–10 minutes until the soft cast sets.

79

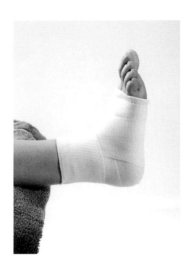

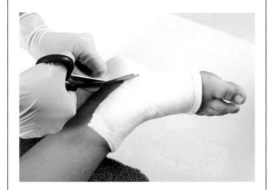

11 Soft cast splint may be left on for several days or weeks depending on the clinical indication. It may get wet without being damaged.

12 If soft cast is to be used as a reusable splint it is possible to cut it off with blunt nose scissors, using a cut on the medial side of the ankle to remove it.

13 Trim any rough edges of the soft cast splint to suit the patient's comfort.

14 Puncture holes on the medial side and use a shoelace to tie the soft cast splint edges together when worn.

Reassessment

○ Patient comfort and symptoms at rest.
○ Circulation in foot and toes.
○ Gait.
○ Provocative movements with or without shoes on.

Follow-up

○ Socks and shoes may be worn over the splint.
○ Splint may be left on for a few days.
○ Splint may be removed with blunt nose scissors by cutting it on the medial side, anterior to the medial malleolus.

Foot soft cast

Background and rationale

Certain foot conditions may benefit from taping, splinting or bracing as an adjunct to usual management (Meyer et al 2002; Osborne et al 2006). Soft cast in the management of foot conditions may be used (Walters et al 2008) as an alternative to taping when:

- tape has caused an allergic skin reaction
- repeated tape use is not an option
- where added support is required for sports
- after removal of rigid cast immobilisation
- it is preferred by the patient.

Evidence

- Walters et al (2008) found that the use of soft cast had an effect on plantar pressures and could be considered as an alternative management approach to controlling foot pronation (Level IV).

Material

- Soft cast material 5 cm or 7.5 cm width.
- Cotton 7.5 cm stockinet to be worn under soft cast.
- Soft dense foam for padding if necessary.
- Plastic gloves.
- Ambient temperature water in a small bowl.
- Blunt nose scissors for trimming and/or removing.
- One small shoe lace if it is to be a reusable splint.

Patient position

- Patient seated or supine on a treatment bed, with the foot over the edge of the bed.

Therapist position

- Standing or seated in front of the foot of the patient. Ensure all materials are within easy reach.

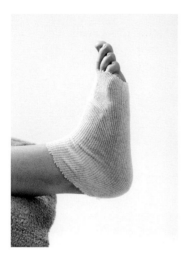

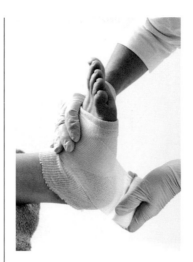

1 Measure, cut and apply 7.5 cm stockinet to the foot.
3 Put plastic gloves on.

4 Open 7.5 cm soft cast tape and roll out like a bandage, applying from the base of the toes at the foot, distal to proximal in figure of 8s, around foot while ensuring there is no tension.
5 Finish just below the malleoli.
6 Overlap each previous layer by half the width of the new layer.
7 When soft cast application is finished, wet hands in cold water and start moulding the splint, pressing around all the bony prominences firmly.
8 Trim soft cast splint to the level of the metatarsophalangeal (MTP) joints, so toe flexion and extension is not impaired.
9 Trim soft cast splint around the ankle so ankle dorsiflexion and plantarflexion is not impaired.
10 Wait a few minutes until the soft cast sets.

80

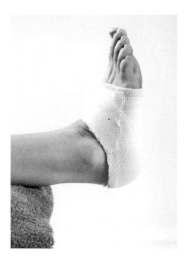

11 Soft cast splint may be left on for a few days or several weeks depending on the clinical indication. It may get wet without being damaged.

12 If soft cast is to be used as a reusable splint it is possible to remove it by cutting it off first.

13 Trim any rough edges of the soft cast splint to suit the patient's comfort.

14 Puncture holes on the dorsal side and use a shoelace to tie the soft cast splint edges together when worn. Tape may also be used to join the splint edges together.

Reassessment
○ Patient comfort and symptoms at rest.
○ Circulation in foot and toes.
○ Gait.
○ Provocative movements with or without shoes on.

Follow-up
○ Socks and shoes may be worn over the splint.
○ Splint may be left on for a couple of days.
○ Splint may be removed with blunt nose scissors by cutting it on the dorsal side.

REFERENCES

Edwards, G S, Jr, DeLee, J C (1984) Ankle diastasis without fracture. Foot Ankle, 4(6): 305–12.

Kerkhoffs, G M, Rowe, B H, Assendelft, W J, Kelly, K, Struijs, P A, van Dijk, C N (2002) Immobilisation and functional treatment for acute lateral ankle ligament injuries in adults. Cochrane Database Systematic Review, (3): CD003762.

Khan, K S, Grufferty, A, Gallagher, O, Moore, D P, Fogarty, E, Dowling, F (2007) A randomized trial of 'soft cast' for distal radius buckle fractures in children. Acta Orthopaedica Belgica, 73(5): 594–7.

Meyer, J, Kulig, K, Landal, R (2002) Differential diagnosis and treatment of subcalcaneal heel pain: a case report. Journal of Orthopaedic & Sports Physical Therapy, 32(3): 114–22.

Neugebauer, H, Fasching, G, Wallenbock, E (1995) Experiences with using the soft cast in injuries of the fibular ligament of the upper ankle joint. Unfallchirurg, 98(9): 489–92.

Osborne, H R, Allison, G T, Hanna, C (2006) Treatment of plantar fasciitis by low dye taping and iontophoresis: short term results of a double blinded, randomised, placebo controlled clinical trial of dexamethasone and acetic acid — commentary. British Journal of Sports Medicine, 40(6): 545–9.

Schuren, J (1994) 3M Working with Soft Cast: a manual on semi-rigid immobilisation. Minnesota Mining & Manufacturing, Minnesota.

Simpson, K J, Cravens, S, Higbie, E, Theodorou, C, DelRey, P (1999) A comparison of the sport stirrup, malleoloc, and Swede-o ankle orthoses for the foot-ankle kinematics of a rapid lateral movement. International Journal of Sports Medicine, 20(6): 396–402.

Walters, J L, Lange, B S, Chipchase, L S (2008) Effect of a low dye application of scotchcast soft cast on peak and mean plantar pressures in subjects with a navicular drop greater than 10 mm. Journal of the American Podiatric Medical Association, 98(6): 457–65.

Appendix 1 Summary of the literature relating to techniques described in Chapters 4, 5 and 6 (alphabetical by author)

In this appendix the levels of evidence follow those described by the Australian National Health and Medical Research Council (NHMRC). As this document does not ascribe a category level for papers without a research component, such as clinical reports, literature reviews, or anecdotal descriptions, papers falling into these categories are described here as clinical reports.

Reference	Design	Body area	Level of evidence (NHMRC)	Subjects
Alexander et al (2003) *Manual Therapy*, 8(1): 37–41	Cohort	Upper and lower trapezius	IV	18 healthy subjects
Bartold et al (2009) *Journal of Science and Medicine in Sport*, 12(suppl 1): S74–S75.	Cadaveric study	Foot	IV	7 fresh intact cadaveric limbs
Bennell et al (2006) *Journal of Orthopaedic Research*, 9: 1854–60.	Randomised within-subject study	Knee	IV	12 currently asymptomatic subjects but with a history of patellofemoral pain
Cowan et al (2006) *British Journal of Sports Medicine*, 40(1): 30–4	Randomised cross-over trial	Knee	III-2	10 subjects with PFPS, plus 12 asymptomatic controls

Intervention and/or taping technique	Outcome measures	Author's conclusions	Comments
Scapula taping consisting of a single strip underwrap tape with an overlying strip of rigid tape applied from the spine of the scapula extending to the lower trapezius muscle	Surface EMG with calculation of the amplitude of the H reflex	Rigid tape decreased the amplitude of the trapezius H reflex by a mean of 22%. This inhibition was not sustained when the tape was removed	No standardisation or monitoring of the tape pressure during application. Asymptomatic subjects
Antipronation taping that inverted the rear foot, everted the forefoot and plantarflexed the 1st ray	Longitudinal strain of the plantar fascia was measured by microstrain gauges	Low dye type taping reduces strain on the plantar fascia compared to no taping	
Subjects performed slow walking, fast walking and stair-climbing tasks with McConnell type patellofemoral tape applied	VMO and VL onset was measured by EMG, stance phase peak knee flexion by 3D motion analysis and peak ground reaction force by force plate	Tape did not affect the onset of timing of VMO or VL. Therapeutic tape led to significant increases in peak knee flexion	No control group
All subjects performed a stair-climbing task with 3 test conditions, no tape, medially directed patella tape and a placebo vertically directed tape	EMG of vastus medialis obliquus (VMO) and vastus lateralis (VL); visual analogue scale (VAS)	Medially directed tape significantly reduced pain. Therapeutic and placebo tape did not alter EMG activity. Pain reduction due to tape is not due to alteration of vasti activity	Comparative trial, randomisation was only within groups

Crossley et al (2009) *Journal of Science and Medicine in Sport*, 12 (suppl 1): S68	Comparative study with a concurrent control group	Knee	III-2	14 subjects with patellofemoral joint osteoarthritis and 14 age matched controls
Fagan & Delahunt (2008) *British Journal of Sports Medicine*, 42(10): 789–95	Systematic review of papers related to the treatment of patellofemoral pain syndrome (PFPS)	Knee	I	Included studies were grouped into 4 sections: (1) hip joint musculature in PFPS; (2) quadriceps muscle imbalance in PFPS; (3) the effects of taping on quadriceps muscle activation in PFPS; (4) open versus closed kinetic chain exercises in PFPS
Franettovich et al (2008) *Medicine and Science in Sports and Exercise*, 40(4): 593–600	Laboratory study; clinical investigation	Ankle	IV	5 asymptomatic subjects with reduced medial longitudinal arch height
Greig et al (2008) *Manual Therapy*, 13(3): 249–57	Cohort	Shoulder, thoracic spine	IV	15 women with osteoporotic fractures of the thoracic spine
Hess (2000) *Manual Therapy*, 5(2): 63–7	Descriptive paper	Shoulder	Clinical report	Not applicable
Hinman et al (2003) *British Medical Journal*, 327 (7407): 135	Single blind randomised controlled trial	Knee	II	87 participants randomised to three groups. Inclusion: clinical and radiological signs of osteoarthritis (OA) as per American College of Radiology criteria. Exclusion: allergy to tape, knee joint replacement, body mass index (BMI) > 38

Patellofemoral taping with medial glide, tilt, and fat pad deloading	MR images of the knee; VAS.	In the symptomatic group patella taping was associated with a significant reduction in lateral patella displacement and also a mean reduction of 15 mm on the VAS	
Varying interventions, most unique to each study in the review but aimed at improving pain and symptoms in PFPS	Varying outcome measures were used in the different papers. The reviewers rated the studies for quality using the Physiotherapy Evidence Database (PEDro) scale.	1 No RCTs were identified that support the use of hip joint strengthening in PFPS 2 Physiotherapy treatment programs appear to be effective for improving quadriceps muscle imbalances 3 More studies are needed to determine the efficacy of patella taping 4 Open and closed kinetic chain exercises are both appropriate in the treatment of PFPS	Various limitations within some or all of the studies identified in the review
Augmented low dye taping technique and walked on treadmill with tape for 10 minutes	Medial longitudinal arch height and EMG activity of tibialis anterior and posterior and peroneus longus	Increase mean arch height (12.9% (6.5–19.3; $p = 0.005$) and reduction in EMG peak and average activity of tibialis anterior and posterior	The participants were asymptomatic
Tape applied bilaterally to improve scapula retraction and thoracic kyphosis	Angle of thoracic kyphosis; EMG	Tape produced a greater reduction in thoracic kyphosis compared to control tape and no tape	No control group
Not applicable	Not applicable	Tape can be used to address humeral head position	Anecdotal evidence only
Patellofemoral tape comprising glide and tilt of the patella, plus patella fat pad unloading tape	VAS, Likert scale, Western Ontario and MacMaster OA index, SF 36	73% of the therapeutic tape group reported improvement in pain and disability, versus 49% in the control tape and 10% in the no tape group	Short duration of the trial. Participants were not able to be blinded

Jamali et al (2004) *Journal of Sports Rehabilitation*, 13: 228–43	Case series	Foot	IV	20 subjects (6 male, 14 female) with plantar fasciitis
Keet et al (2007) *Physiotherapy*, 93(1): 45–52	Placebo-controlled clinical control with randomisation of interventions	Knee	III-1	15 subjects with PFPS pain, 20 asymptomatic subjects
Khan et al (2007) *Acta Orthopaedica Belgica*, 73(5): 594–7	Randomised controlled trial	Wrist	II	117 children with stable fractures of the distal radius
Kilbreath et al (2006) *Australian Journal of Physiotherapy*, 52(1): 53–6	Case series	Hip	IV	15 stroke patients with impaired gait
Macgregor et al (2005) *Journal of Orthopaedic Research*, 23(2): 351–8	Experimental study with pre test post test	Knee	IV	8 subjects with patellofemoral pain of anterior knee pain > 3 months
Marin (1998) *Archives of Physical Medicine & Rehabilitation*, 79(10): 1226–30	Case series	Shoulder	IV	14 patients in a military setting with symptoms of thoracic nerve palsy of 3 months or greater duration

Patients with symptoms of plantar fasciitis were treated with a taping technique designed to reduce mid-foot pronation and the windlass effect	VAS. Measurements of calcaneal and tibial position using an inclinometer, and also of navicular height using an indexed card	Taping that reduces pronation reduces the strain on the plantar fascia caused by the windlass effect	No control group or patient or operator blinding
Pain, quadriceps force and EMG were measured during maximal quads testing with 3 different test conditions of no tape, placebo tape and medial tape	VAS, isometric and isokinetic force output, EMG analysis	Tape did not significantly decrease pain or increase force output, but did significantly enhance the efficiency of VMO activity in both groups	Relevance of the force measures used limits the usefulness of the findings of this study
After randomisation into 2 different groups, children with stable distal radius fractures were treated either with a rigid cast or with soft cast. In both groups the cast was worn for 3 weeks	Fracture healing, reported problems with the cast	Both groups had full recovery. Only one patient in the soft cast group reported problems with the cast compared with 5 patients in the rigid cast group	Outcome measures not clearly described
All subjects were tested with gluteal taping compared to no taping and sham taping	Hip extension and step length both measured at 2 different walking speeds	Hip extension increased significantly at both walking speeds with gluteal taping. Step length on the unaffected side was increased significantly at both walking speeds	No control group
Taping on the patella, subjects maintained a sustained contraction and stretch was applied in 3 directions	Measured EMG activity of single motor units in vastus medialis obliquus (VMO)	Taping causing skin stretch over VMO may increase motor unit firing rate in VMO	
A brace designed to reduce scapula winging	Manual muscle tests, patient satisfaction questionnaire	The brace increased strength as identified in the manual muscle tests. Patients reported decreased pain and subjective feelings of increased strength	No control group. Validity of manual muscle tests as an outcome measure

McCarthy Persson, Fleming, Caulfield (2009) The effect of a vastus lateralis tape on muscle activity during stair climbing. *Manual Therapy*, 14(3): 330-7	Case series with pre test and post test	Vastus lateralis	IV	25 asymptomatic subjects
McConnell (1986) The management of chondromalacia patellae: a long-term solution. *Australian Journal of Physiotherapy*, 32: 215-23	Case series	Knee (patella)	IV	35 participants (12-37 years — 20 females and 15 males) with a diagnosis of chandromalacia patellae
McConnell (2000) *Journal of Science and Medicine in Sport*, 3(3): 325-34	Descriptive paper with three case reports	Shoulder	Clinical report	Three case studies each involving one patient each. For the shoulder case study a volleyball player with glenohumeral (GH) instability
McConnell and McIntosh (2009) *Clinical Journal of Sport Medicine*, 19(2): 90-4	Case series with pre test and post test	Shoulder	IV	21 tennis players, 11 male, 10 female (asymptomatic)
Moiler et al (2006) *Journal of Orthopaedic & Sports Physical Therapy*, 36(9): 661-8	Prospective non-randomised controlled clinical trial	Ankle	III-3	125 male basketball players, age range 13-23 years
Morin et al (1997) *Journal of Sports Rehabilitation* 6(4): 309-18	Case series with pre test and post test	Shoulder — scapula stability	IV	10 uninjured subjects

EMG collected during 3 conditions: no tape (untaped), control tape (no tension) and tensioned tape (VL inhibitory taping application perpendicular to the muscle)	Normalised integrated EMG (IEMG) collected from vastus lateralis (VL), vastus medialis obliquus (VMO), biceps femoris (BF) and soleus muscles during stair climbing	VL IEMG significantly decreased in tape and control subjects ($p < 0.05$) in initial stance phase during both stair ascent and descent. No significant differences ($p > 0.05$) were seen in the other tested muscles	The study was performed on asymptomatic subjects
Patella tape for patella repositioning plus exercises	Pain	83% no pain after 3–8 treatments	No standardisation of diagnosis, outcome measures and no control. Landmark study that others were based on
In the shoulder case study a taping technique designed to improve position and stability of the head of humerus	Symptoms of pain and GH instability, a functional volleyball task	Tape can be used to address humeral head position	Lack of clear outcome measures. Sample size
Humeral head repositioning with tape	Glenohumeral ROM measured by goniometry	Tape resulted in a significant increase in both GH external and internal rotation	Generalisability of the results is questionable due to the narrow age range and adolescent population
Fibula repositioning tape (FRT) as described by Mulligan	Injury incidence data. Ankle injury severity scale	Subjects who used the FRT sustained significantly less ankle injuries than the control group. FRT appears to be more effective in reducing ankle injuries than other 'traditional' taping methods	Lack of blinding and randomisation. The control condition was not a true control as some of the athletes in this group used other preventative measures such as traditional taping or bracing
A taping technique applied with the goal of decreasing upper trapezius activity	EMG recordings from upper, middle and lower trapezius	Tape decreased upper trapezius activity with a commensurate increase in middle and lower trapezium activity	No control group. No blinding of subjects or assessors

Morrissey (2000) *Journal of Bodywork and Movement Therapies*, 4: 189–94	Two single case reports (descriptive paper)	Shoulder	Clinical report	Not applicable
O'Brien & Vicenzino (1998) *Manual Therapy*, 3(2): 78–84	Single case study	Ankle	Level IV	2 male subjects
O'Leary et al (2002) *Manual Therapy*, 7(3): 150–3	Randomised, single blind placebo-controlled repeated measures study	Thoracic spine	IV	24 asymptomatic subjects
Overington et al (2006) *NZ Journal of Physiotherapy*, 34(2): 66–80	Systematic review of papers related to the treatment of PFPS	Knee	I	21 randomised controlled clinical trials and clinical trials were reviewed
Poolman et al (2005) *Cochrane Database of Systematic Reviews.* Online: http://www.mrw.interscience.wiley.com/cochrane/clsysrev/articles/CD003210/frame.html	Systematic review	Fifth metacarpal fractures	I	Variable between the reviewed studies

Not specified	None	Tape can enhance shoulder proprioception, possibly through stimulation of mechanoreceptors in the skin	Anecdotal opinion only
A Mulligan type mobilisation with movement technique for the ankle was followed with a taping technique designed to maintain the posterior glide of the distal fibula	Modified Kaikkonnen test, range of dorsiflexion and inversion, VAS	Improvement in both subjects occurred that appeared to be more than usually attributable to natural improvement	Single case study design limits generalisation of the findings
All 24 subjects were assessed for thoracic spine pressure pain threshold before and after 3 different conditions of a deloading tape technique, a sham tape and no tape	Pressure pain threshold at the T7 spinous process	There was no significant difference between pressure pain thresholds in this asymptomatic group. However, tape may be useful to deload or inhibit injured tissues in the thoracic spine of symptomatic subjects	Subjects were asymptomatic
Varying interventions, most unique to each study in the review but aimed at improving pain and symptoms in PFPS	Varying outcome measures were used in the different papers. The reviewers rated the included studies for quality using the PEDro scale	Patella taping appears to decrease pain in the short term, may be beneficial in the long term in conjunction with other physiotherapy treatments, and can alter VMO activity	The limitations of the individual studies included in the review
Variable between the reviewed studies	Variable between the reviewed studies	Tape is a valid option for treatment of closed 5th metacarpal fractures	

Prosser (1995) *Australian Journal of Physiotherapy*, 41(1): 41–6	Descriptive paper with two single case reports, one involving tape	Wrist — triangular fibrocartilaginous complex (TFCC) injury	Clinical report	1 female, 23 years old, with a TFCC injury
Rarick et al (1962) *Journal of Bone and Joint Surgery*, 44(6): 1183–90	Case series	Ankle	IV	5 male subjects 21–28 years old
Rettig et al (1997) *The American Journal of Sports Medicine*, 25(1): 96–8	Cohort	Finger and wrist	IV	25 American football players. Age and gender not specified
Selkowitz et al (2007) *Journal of Orthopaedic & Sports Physical Therapy*, 37(11): 694–702	Cohort	Shoulder	IV	21 subjects with shoulder pain (11 male, 10 female
Shamus & Shamus (1997) *Journal of Orthopaedic & Sports Physical Therapy*, 25(6): 390–4	Two case reports	Shoulder–AC joint	Clinical report	2 subjects with grade III AC joint separation injuries
Stoddard & Johnson (2000) *Journal of Sports Chiropractic & Rehabilitation*, 14(4): 118–28	Single case report	Shoulder–AC joint	Clinical report	1 subject diagnosed with a grade I AC joint separation injury

Ulnar carpal taping, a wrist support brace and strengthening exercises	Subjective assessment of pain and function, grip strength	Tape can be used as an adjunct to treatment in cases of carpal instability	Treatments were applied concurrently so whether the patients' improvement can be attributed in part or in full to any of the individual components of the treatment program cannot be determined from this study
Compared 4 different taping techniques for the ankle	Resistance to inversion and plantar flexion as measured with a cable tensiometer	Basket weave taping with stirrups and heel lock was more supportive than the normal basket weave with no heel lock. Up to 40% of the support was lost after 10 minutes of vigorous exercise	Force measurements were only calculated at one position. Small sample size, no randomisation or blinding
Self-taping of wrist and fingers — technique not described and not standardised	Grip strength dynamometer	Un-taped dominant hand significantly stronger than taped dominant hand (Mean grip 142.7 vs 137.8 pounds [$p = 0.02$])	Taping technique not standardised
Scapula taping consisting of a single strip underwrap tape with an overlying strip of rigid tape applied over the upper trapezius of the affected side, extending from the clavicle to the lower trapezius	EMG. Functional reaching task	Tape was associated with decreased upper trapezius and increased lower trapezius EMG activity during shoulder elevation and abduction	The differences while significant were small
A taping technique designed to reduce pain and allow effective exercise to be performed	Verbal analogue pain scale. ROM measured by a goniometer. Manual muscle strength tests	Both patients reported decreased pain. ROM and strength as assessed by the therapists both improved	Validity and accuracy of the outcome measures
Chiropractic spinal manipulation plus supportive taping for the AC joint	Patients' subjective reports of pain and ability to perform activities of daily living	Tape added stability to the shoulder which decreased pain and allowed earlier rehabilitation	Validity and accuracy of the outcome measures. Two diverse interventions used concurrently

Timm (1985) *Journal of Orthopaedic & Sports Physical Therapy*, 6(6): 334–42	Descriptive paper	Thumb — MCP joint	Clinical report	Not applicable
Tobin & Robinson (2000) *Physiotherapy*, 86(4): 174–83	Same-subject re-test report	Thigh/knee	IV	18 asymptomatic subjects (11 female, 7 male). Inclusion and/or exclusion criteria not specified.
Vaes et al (1985) *Journal of Orthopaedic & Sports Physical Therapy*, 7(3): 110–14	Comparative radiological study	Ankle	IV	51 athletes from various sports
Vicenzino et al (2003) *Journal of Orthopaedic & Sports Physical Therapy*, 33(7): 400–7	Single-blind, placebo-controlled, randomised, cross-over study	Elbow – lateral epicondylalgia	IV	16 subjects with chronic lateral epicondylalgia
Vicenzino et al (2005) *British Journal of Sports Medicine*, 39(12): 935–43	Repeated measures study	Foot	IV	17 subjects (5 male, 12 female) assympatomatic, but with a navicular drop greater than 10 mm

Thumb spica taping technique for 1st MCP joint	None	Tape can be used as an adjunct in the management of ulnar instability of the MCP joint	Anecdotal opinion only. No comparative research or functional outcome measures
Unloading tape was placed on the upper vastus lateralis and a stair-climbing task was performed. Placebo tape and no tape conditions were also tested	EMG of VMO and VL	VMO and VL activity was significantly decreased with the taping technique. VMO and VL activity was increased with the placebo taping technique	Asymptomatic subjects only. No control group
A varus stress was applied to the tibiotalar joint using an apparatus that allowed control over force and range of motion. Subjects were tested without any external support, with an elastic bandage applied, and with a basket weave taping technique using rigid strapping tape both before a 30 minute activity test including jumping and running exercises	X-ray of the ankle joint in the various test conditions	Rigid taping produced the greatest decrease in talar tilt angle. After the 30 minute activity program the reduction in talar tilt was still highly significant	Talar tilt ankle may give information about the support to the calcaneo-fibular ligament, but probably less so for the more frequently injured anterior talo-fibular ligament.
'Diamond' taping technique designed to reduce load on painful forearm extensors	Pain-free grip strength with a dynamometer, pressure pain threshold	Pain-free grip strength was significantly improved by 24% from baseline ($p = 0.028$). Pressure pain threshold improved by 19% but this was not statistically significant	No separate control group
The effect of the standard low dye taping technique on foot posture was compared with the augmented low dye taping	Vertical navicular height during standing, walking and after 20 minutes of jogging was assessed by a measure of medial longitudinal arch (MLA) height as determined from video	The augmented low dye taping is superior to standard low dye for increasing MLA height in all 3 test conditions	

Vicenzino & Wright (1995) *Manual Therapy*, 1(1): 30-5		Single case report	IV	1 subject with lateral epicondylalgia
Walters et al (2008) *Journal of the American Podiatric Medical Association*, 98(6): 457-65		Same-subject, repeated measures study	IV	32 subjects, age range 18–35 years, with a navicular drop of greater than 10 mm

A sustained lateral glide of the elbow held in place with tape	VAS, pressure algometer, grip strength dynamometer	Pain-free grip strength and pain was reduced with a lateral glide and taping	Only 1 subject
Barefoot walking was compared with walking with a low dye type technique made with soft cast applied	Plantar pressure as measured by a force plate	Soft cast significantly affected plantar pressures. Soft cast may provide an alternative to current management techniques in controlling foot pronation and reducing symptoms of lower-limb abnormalities	No control group

Appendix 2 Patient Information Sheet

Date
_____

The main aim of this taping technique is to
_____

_____

As a precaution to taping it is important that you inform me if you have any of the following conditions:
○ skin allergy or sensitivity to tape
○ open wounds
○ skin infections or conditions such as dermatitis, eczema
○ fragile or sensitive skin in the area to be taped, which is prone to tears and bruising
○ circulatory conditions — bleeding or clotting disorders
○ loss of sensation, pins and needles or numbness around the area to be taped
○ peripheral vascular disease
○ peripheral neuropathies
○ diabetes
○ prolonged use of steroid or blood thinning (anticoagulant) medication.

Adhesive tape may cause skin irritation to some people. With prolonged or repeated use of tape application and removal, adhesive tapes may possibly cause adhesive contact dermatitis or irritant contact dermatitis in some people. Prior to applying tape,

I would like to ask you:
○ Do you have any known allergy to tape, band-aids or other adhesive material?
○ If you are not certain and in order to test if you have a tendency to be sensitive to the adhesive materials used in rigid tapes, I would like to apply a small 2 cm strip of tape for 20 minutes near the area to be treated to see if you demonstrate any skin reaction, redness, itchiness or irritability to tape.
○ If you develop adhesive or irritant contact dermatitis during or after tape application, the tape and any adhesive residue should be removed completely, and cold water applied to cool the area. If the irritation does not settle, is painful, or the skin has broken down, you should visit your local doctor or hospital for medical assessment and management.

POST-TAPING PRECAUTIONS AND WARNINGS

During and after each application of a taping technique I would like to ensure that:

1 the taping technique is comfortable and you have no feelings of restriction, tightness or pain

2 you are not experiencing any pins and needles, numbness or other symptoms of impaired circulation.

After you leave this practice and at any time it is important to be aware that you may leave the tape on for up to 48 hours. The tape can become wet if you wish to swim or shower with it on. However, you must ensure the tape is adequately dry prior to being covered. If at any time you are experiencing:

○ additional discomfort

○ increase in any of your symptoms

○ feelings of pins and needles or numbness at the site of the tape, around the area of the tape, or below the area being taped

○ feelings of skin itchiness or irritability under the tape

○ skin colour changes around the tape such as pallor, redness or blueness

○ skin temperature changes such as a feeling of coldness or hot to touch, and/or

○ increased swelling around the tape

you must remove the tape immediately. The tape can be removed by folding it back on itself as shown to you, and using a pair of scissors to cut the tape off after lifting away from your body. The tape can also be removed using eucalyptus oil if you have no allergy to this. If you have any concerns regarding the application and removal of this taping technique please feel free to contact me.

Do you understand this warning?   Yes/No

Do you have any questions?

_____

_____

_____

_____

_____

_____

If you understand what has been explained to you and you are happy to proceed, please sign below.

Name

_____

Signature

_____

Therapist name

_____

Therapist signature

_____

Date

_____

Index

ICD *see* irritant contact dermatitis
iliotibial band (ITB)
    deloading 132–3
    friction syndrome deloading 134–5
    tenderness 115
    see also hip joint and buttock
Iliotibial band friction syndrome (ITBFS) 134
inclinometer measure 4–5
inferior tibiofibular joint subluxation 162–3
inferiorly subluxed HOH 64–7
    see also shoulder joint
informed consent 35
interphalangeal toe joints 196–7
irritant contact dermatitis (ICD) 22, 34
ITB *see* iliotibial band
ITBFS *see* Iliotibial band friction syndrome

Jaylastic 21
'Jersey finger' 105–6
    see also hand, thumb and finger

Kinesio® 20
kinetic type taping research 20
knee joint
    anterior cruciate ligament (ACL) injury
        144–6
    facilitating tibial rotation 146–7
    iliotibial band friction syndrome deloading
        134–5
    lateral collateral ligament 141–3
    medial collateral ligament 138–40
    Pes anserinus bursitis/tendinopathy
        deloading 136–7
    preventing knee hyperextension 144–6
knowledge of anatomy 6

lateral collateral ligament (LCL) injury, knee
    141–3
lateral epicondylalgia (LE) 74
    diamond deloading for 75
    reinforcing lateral glide for 78–9
    wrist extensor muscle deloading for 76–7
lateral meniscus injury, knee 141–3
LCL *see* lateral collateral ligament
LE *see* lateral epicondylalgia
Leukoplast 21
levels of evidence 3
literature review 12, 27
    ankle sprain prevention 26
    deloading and/or unloading 18–19
    effects on oedema 29
    elbow lateral epicondylalgia 24–5
    kinetic type taping 20
    pain reduction 13–17
    patellofemoral pain 25–6
    plantar fasciitis 26–7
    proprioception enhancement 17–18
    psychological effects 19
    scapular and shoulder 23–4
    side-effects of tape 22
    summary 240–55
    tape and adhesive characteristics 21–2
    VMO and VL research 16, 148
long thoracic nerve palsy 56
    see also scapula position
low dye foot anti-pronation technique 14, 183–4
    augmented 185–6
lower trapezius muscle facilitation 52–3
lumbar spine
    support 212–13
    thoracolumbar fascial deloading
        214–15

zygapophyseal (facet) joint deloading
    216–17
lumbrical grip 7

magnetic resonance imaging (MRI) 13, 25
'mallet finger' 103–4
    see also hand, thumb and finger
materials for taping 36–7
McConnell, Jenny 11
MCL *see* medial collateral ligament
MCP *see* metacarpophalangeal
MDI *see* multidirectional instability
mechanical effects of tape 13–15
medial collateral ligament (MCL) injury, knee
    138–40
medial longitudinal arch (MLA) height 14,
    26–7
    low dye taping for 182–3
medial meniscus injury, knee 138–40
medial tibial stress syndrome (MTSS) 180
Medline 12
Mefix 21
metacarpal fractures 98–9
    see also hand, thumb and finger
metacarpophalangeal (MCP) joint 94, 229
Micropore tape 21
MLA *see* medial longitudinal arch
MRI *see* magnetic resonance imaging
MTSS *see* medial tibial stress syndrome
mobilisation with movement (MWM)
    techniques 14–15, 19
        elbow lateral glide 78
        inferior tibiofibular joint subluxation 162
        superior tibiofibular joint subluxation 160
        tibial external or internal rotation 146
        toe interphalangeal joints 196